£19·99

Anxiety

EDUCATION CENTRE LIBRARY
FURNESS GENERAL HOSPITAL
BARROW-IN-FURNESS

YOUR QUESTIONS ANSWERED

D1375337

Commissioning Editor: Ellen Green
Project Development and Management: Fiona Conn
Design: George Ajayi, Jayne Jones, Keith Kail
Illustrator: Evi Antoniou

Anxiety

YOUR QUESTIONS ANSWERED

Trevor Turner
BA MB BS MD FRCPsych
Consultant Psychiatrist and Clinical Director, Homerton Hospital and St
Bartholomew's Hospital, London, UK

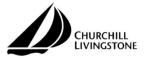
CHURCHILL
LIVINGSTONE

EDINBURGH LONDON NEW YORK PHILADELPHIA ST LOUIS SYDNEY TORONTO 2003

CHURCHILL LIVINGSTONE
An imprint of Elsevier Science Limited

616.8522
Tur

© 2003, Elsevier Science Limited. All rights reserved.

The right of Trevor Turner to be identified as author of this work has
been asserted by him in accordance with the Copyright, Designs
and Patents Act 1988

No part of this publication may be reproduced, stored in a retrieval
system, or transmitted in any form or by any means, electronic,
mechanical, photocopying, recording or otherwise, without either the
prior permission of the publishers (Permissions Manager,
Elsevier Science Ltd, Robert Stevenson House, 1-3 Baxter's Place,
Leith Walk, Edinburgh EH1 3AF), or a licence permitting restricted
copying in the United Kingdom issued by the Copyright Licensing
Agency, 90 Tottenham Court Road, London W1T 4LP.

First published 2003

ISBN 0 443 07294 9   SMC

British Library Cataloguing in Publication Data
A catalogue record for this book is available from the British Library

Library of Congress Cataloging in Publication Data
A catalog record for this book is available from the Library of Congress

Note
Medical knowledge is constantly changing. As new information becomes
available, changes in treatment, procedures, equipment and the use of
drugs become necessary. The authors and the publishers have taken care
to ensure that the information given in this text is accurate and up to
date. However, readers are strongly advised to confirm that the
information, especially with regard to drug usage, complies with the latest
legislation and standards of practice.

**ELSEVIER
SCIENCE**
your source for books,
journals and multimedia
in the health sciences
www.elsevierhealth.com

The
publisher's
policy is to use
**paper manufactured
from sustainable forests**

Printed in China

Contents

Preface

This book is aimed at providing practical and realistic answers to a series of, literally, worrying questions. Anxiety disorders pervade so many areas of health service practice, both in primary and hospital care. They are poorly understood, and are often downgraded as problems in living rather than real illnesses. The aim of this book is to show that they can be understood; that there are ways of dealing with them that are logical, and not necessarily demanding of super-specialist resources; and that GPs can take the lead in developing treatments.

A GP with a list of say 2500 patients, given the general prevalence rates of anxiety disorders, especially that elusive category of 'mixed anxiety and depression', is going to have over 200 patients with these conditions on the books. While no one would suggest that they can all be, somehow, miraculously 'cured' by the right combination of modern medications and perhaps cognitive or behavioural psychotherapy, there remains enormous potential for reducing morbidity and improving the quality of people's lives. It is also an area where a range of other professionals, as well as voluntary groups, can be usefully employed, and where patients themselves can take on caring roles.

In this sense, the management of anxiety is very much part of modern medicine, seeing the doctor as part of a team, clinically responsible but prepared to delegate tasks to community nurses, psychologists, social workers, or patient user groups. The combination of current initiatives in terms of the National Service Framework and the development of Primary Care Trusts should give just the kind of impetus that this treatment approach needs.

The heart of this book derives from a large number of patient-generated questions, both personal and from lists of patient groups, as well as from 15 years of answering GPs' questions over the phone, in their surgeries, and in numerous casual contacts ranging from the squash court to the supermarket. The need to avoid over-technical language, a particular curse unfortunately of some forms of psychiatric practice, and the need to see anxiety as very much a psycho-physiological state (not just a state of mind) underlie the book's approach. It is designed to be both accessible and honest – the author does not consider that if only practitioners were competent enough then all anxiety disorders would be curable. It is also designed to make it easier to accentuate the positive in managing these conditions, the 'cure' of which will undoubtedly be the basis for several Nobel Prizes in Medicine one day.

This book would not have been possible to write without the contribution of the thousands (literally) of patients, who have 'patiently' clarified to me the nature of their symptoms, how they try to deal with them, what has been helpful and what has not been helpful. Colleagues and friends at Homerton University Hospital, who have given advice and comments, and many heroic GP colleagues – who are in the front line of anxiety management, so to speak – also need to be thanked for the numerous thoughtful comments and conversations, over the years, that have helped clarify problems and useful approaches.

The brilliant typing and word organizational skills of Jon Flint, who has dealt so heroically with a manuscript of Protean changeability, also need to be acknowledged.

TT

How to use this book

The *Your Questions Answered* series aims to meet the information needs of GPs and other primary care professionals who care for patients with chronic conditions. It is designed to help them work with patients and their families, providing effective, evidence-based care and management.

The books are in an accessible question and answer format, with detailed contents lists at the beginning of every chapter and a complete index to help find specific information.

ICONS

Icons are used in the book to identify particular types of information:

 highlights important information

 highlights side-effect information.

PATIENT QUESTIONS

At the end of relevant chapters there are sections of frequently asked patient questions, with easy-to-understand answers aimed at the non-medical reader. These questions are also listed at the end of the book.

Anxiety: an introduction

1

1.1 What is normal anxiety?

Normal anxiety is the sympathetic nervous arousal that precedes and is part of the 'fight or flight' response. It reflects the psychological and physical state required to deal with an emergency, and is a normal way of reacting to a number of demanding situations. The ability of certain people to shine in a crisis, or of certain athletes to 'psych' themselves up for a big race, is based on the temporary efficiencies of being a bit anxious. Jumping out of the way of an on-rushing cyclist, fielding questions in an interview, or running and catching a cricket ball would be typical examples. Blood flow is increased, thinking is speeded up, muscle power is raised, and reactions are enhanced. It is also probably true to state that very few people are completely un-anxious. Dealing with the humdrum business of life constantly makes demands, with minor fears, social pressures, guilty thoughts and random events breaking the calm or requiring action. Learning to deal with all this can be seen as part of social adaptation, of becoming a real grown-up.

1.2 What is the difference between normal anxiety and morbid ('clinical') anxiety?

There is no difference in the *kind* of symptoms people get, such as an increased heart rate (often perceived as palpitations) or muscle tension, but rather in the *level* and *intensity* of those symptoms. The classic description of the difference lies in the Yerkes–Dodson curve, which shows efficiency increasing with increasing anxiety, until a peak is reached when suddenly it all falls apart (*Fig. 1.1*). Instead of feeling alert you feel panicky; instead of being on your toes you feel muscle pains or cramps; instead of feeling strong and steady you are dominated by feeling weak and tremulous. Furthermore, normal anxiety should have an understandable basis (i.e. someone is pushing you to do something) while morbid anxiety often comes on for no obvious reason, or for a reason that seems silly but cannot be put out of mind. Normal anxiety helps to get things done well; morbid anxiety makes one feel ill. It also has the annoying quality of making people worry as to why they are so worried.

1.3 Can anxiety be helpful or even useful in some situations?

It certainly seems that some people, like top athletes or tennis players, can harness their own psychological state to improve their performance (*see Q. 1.1*). The process of worrying about, for example, an exam, can make sure one gets on with revising, can improve the quality of concentration, and can improve retention of material. Likewise, the usual anxiety reactions, such as being sick or needing to go to the toilet to pass stool, can be helpful ways of making sure that, before you exercise, your gastrointestinal system is cleared out. Increasing blood flow to the limbs can both enhance speed

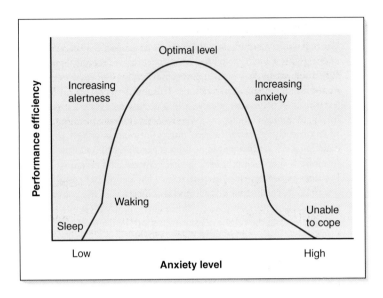

▲

Fig. 1.1 Yerkes–Dodson curve. (From Beers & Berkow 1999, after Yerkes & Dodson 1908)

and power and warm you up, if you like to partake in sports. Not being anxious, by contrast, can leave one 'cold' in terms of dealing with situations, less aware of what is going on, and sluggish in reaction. The over-calm, phlegmatic interviewee, for example, can make an appointments committee feel that he (or she) is not that interested or interesting.

1.4 What is meant by the phrase 'a nervous breakdown'?

This is a commonly used term that has no specific meaning. It probably derived from an attempt to give a formal, somatic label to people panicking, crying, or being upset about a particular experience. Fainting, vomiting, screaming or going into a range of complex gesticulations – depending on a person's age, culture, gender, etc. – have always been part of the response to troubling or fearful events. The term has also been used by doctors in the past to try to avoid using more stigmatizing terms (e.g. schizophrenia); thus it tends to cover a multitude of sins. If patients tell you that they or members of their family have had a 'nervous breakdown' it is worth asking just what in fact happened, and in what circumstances. This can be useful in establishing a family history, or in getting them to talk about particular symptoms.

1.5   Is anxiety more common than it was?

There is no evidence that people are any more anxious than they used to be, although there are constant theories about the 'pressures' of modern life. While formal diagnoses of anxiety disorders, including panic attacks and mixed anxiety/depression, are more commonly made now, a look at the historical literature shows very similar symptoms under a different rubric (e.g. neurasthenia; *see Fig. 1.2*). The resort to personal tranquillizers,

17th C	MELANCHOLY *The Anatomy of Melancholy*	Burton (1621)
18th/19th C	NEUROSIS	Cullen (1803)
	The term 'neurosis' was coined in the 18th century to describe those illnesses reckoned to be due to weakness or abnormality of the nerves, but for which no obvious lesion could be found,* e.g. palpitatio melancholia	
19th C	NERVOUSNESS e.g. 'the vapours'	
	PLATZSCHWINDEL (place dizziness)	Benedikt (1870)
	IRRITABLE HEART	Da Costa (1871)
	AGORAPHOBIA	Westphal (1872)
	CEREBRO-CARDIAC NEUROSIS	Krishaber (1873)
	NEURASTHENIA	Beard (1880)
	ANXIETY NEUROSIS	Freud (1894)
Early 20th C	PSYCHASTHENIA SOLDIER'S HEART NEUROCIRCULATORY ASTHENIA	
Today	PANIC DISORDER GENERALIZED ANXIETY DISORDER	

* This lack of any clear physical abnormality continues to be a problem today, for both sufferers and clinicians.

Fig. 1.2 Historical descriptions of anxiety

EDUCATION CENTRE LIBRARY
FURNESS GENERAL HOSPITAL
BARROW-IN-FURNESS

whether alcohol, tobacco, or calming drugs like opium, has been a commonplace of human society down the ages, particularly urban society. Every generation also experiences a speeding up of life, and there is probably a sense that people do more in one day now (and 'talk' more over their mobile phone or email?) than they used to. They also take less exercise, while completing more tasks (e.g. turning on a tap rather than walking half a mile to and from the water pump) so they have a sense of more going on in their lives. If more is going on, then there is more potential to worry about things.

Furthermore, there is no evidence from research studies that the prevalence of anxiety is increasing. But it does seem to be better recognized in a world where other more serious illnesses (e.g. infections) have been largely eliminated. There is also a wider range of terms used to describe it, whether populist such as 'being stressed up', or technical such as arousability or hypervigilance. The amount of information available about all sorts of common ailments, in magazines, on television and on the Internet, probably makes people think more about their personal symptoms. It is also likely that our sugar and caffeine consumption habits do enhance levels of metabolism and irritability (via a neurophysiological effect), while noise, crowds and information overload add to the potential for 'stress'.

1.6 Is anxiety a problem more in urban and industrialized countries?

There is no evidence that anxiety is commoner in so-called advanced or urban societies, although it may be more apparent. Many people choose to live in the countryside because it is quieter (as in the folk story of the 'town mouse' versus the 'country mouse') and become easily anxious if they have to go to the city. Furthermore, since city life often involves office work rather than physical labour, it is more likely that individuals will have a range of symptoms that might have been eased (at least in part) by the simple efficacies of regular exercise. The current fashion for working out in gyms may be related to this kind of experience. In addition, more advanced societies have reduced rates of physical illnesses such as tuberculosis and anaemia, thus making psychological symptoms more overt. Enhanced expectations of personal comfort, on a day-to-day basis, may also lead individuals to seek medical help, not least because it is likely to be available and quite near at hand.

1.7 How common are anxiety disorders?

The simple answer is that they are not rare, with prevalence rates of between 3% and 10%, depending on how they are defined (*Figs 1.3 and 1.4*). The lifetime prevalence of combined depression/anxiety is between 15% and 20%, while a 1995 household survey in the UK showed figures of about 10% for all anxiety disorders (including panic attacks, phobias, etc.). Anxiety symptoms, singly or in association with other psychological or physical symptoms, probably account for up to a third of all consultations in general practice, and are particularly associated with the 'frequent attender'. Some 50% of new referrals to gastroenterology clinics, for example, turn out to have irritable bowel syndrome, i.e. a significant anxiety component. Likewise some 20% of new referrals to cardiology outpatients are probably anxiety based (due, especially, to palpitations), as are over 50% of new referrals to neurology clinics (headaches, dizziness, etc.). If just half of these could be managed in the GP surgery, think of the impact on outpatient waiting times.

1.8 Are there any particular age groups who seem more prone to anxiety problems?

Much of the reporting on the typical 'anxious' patient can be anecdotal. However, while the incidence of depression is more common in older age groups (the over-60s), first-onset anxiety seems to be something associated

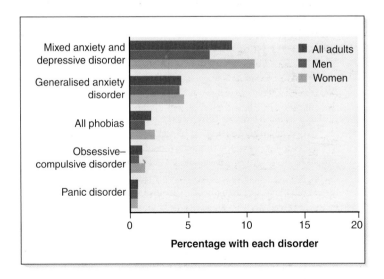

Fig. 1.3 Prevalence of anxiety disorders among adults aged 16–74 in Great Britain. (After Ferriman 2001, with permission of the BMJ Publishing Group.)

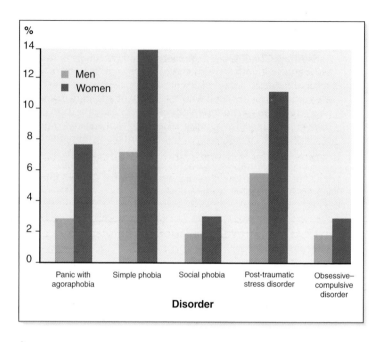

▲

Fig. 1.4 Lifetime rates of various anxiety disorders in men and women from community studies. (From Yonkers 1994)

with the under-40s. It may even be that people learn to adapt as they grow older. Anxiety, with or without panic attacks, typically presents as a problem in the second or third decade, and learning to deal with it at that age involves a greater likelihood of seeking medical advice.

The corollary of this is that later-onset conditions, in one's 40s or 50s, should be more closely investigated. Care should be taken, of course, to ensure that so-called first-onset 'anxiety disorder', in a 45-year-old woman for example, has not actually been around for a long time. Some social factor may lead her to seek advice only after putting up with distressing isolation, perhaps due to agoraphobia, for many years.

1.9 Is clinical anxiety more common in women?

In terms of presentations this does seem to be true, in that women present two to three times more often than men, complaining of anxiety and the typical symptoms thereof (*Figs 1.3 and 1.4*). This reflects the higher attendance rates of women in GP surgeries anyway, but may also reflect a differential presentation in men. Thus, the anxious man may complain of impotence, or stress at work, or other somatic symptoms (e.g. headaches), because of the stigma attached to psychological problems. Alternatively he may present with a drug or alcohol problem, both of these conditions being more prevalent in males. However, conditions like premenstrual tension, or child care problems and marital breakdown, have a greater impact on women; thus the greater likelihood of them having something to feel anxious about. *Table 1.1* summarizes the factors behind the *apparently* greater likelihood of women having anxiety disorders.

1.10   Is anxiety commoner in certain cultural or ethnic groups?

In terms of culture or ethnicity, people who have had frightening experiences as refugees, or as migrants, are more likely to feel affected by their experiences or their sense of social dislocation. The specific problems of post-traumatic stress disorder (*see Q. 5.18*), 'reactive' depression, and even classical 'nostalgia' (i.e. the pain of being far away from one's natural home) can present superficially as just a form of anxiety. The presentation of physical symptoms by patients with a less sophisticated health language – sometimes termed 'health anxiety' – is a particular diagnostic dilemma, but no single ethnic group shows clearly increased rates of formal anxiety disorders.

1.11   Does anxiety commonly lead to other illnesses?

There is some evidence that clinical anxiety is related, in itself, to the development of other disorders. It may underlie a range of associated physical presentations, like irritable bowel syndrome or constant jaw-chewing at night (trismus), which may lead on to secondary conditions. So-called type A personality is associated with enhanced rates of coronary disease, but whether this is causal, or part and parcel, of the same condition is unknown. Thus a common factor (an overactive adrenaline arousal system, for example) may lead to a sense of psychological urgency *and* narrowing of

TABLE 1.1 Are women really more anxious than men?	
Women	Men
Visit the doctor more often	Tend to hide symptoms/avoid the GP
Higher rates of reputed depression	Use work/sport as an outlet
Problems of child care	'Dominant role' protection
Physical disorders such as premenstrual tension or the menopause	Somatize their symptoms ('wind'/'acidity')
Social role → oppression	Act out anxiety via aggression, thus much higher crime/prison rate
Higher rates of smoking	Higher rate of alcohol/drug abuse

coronary arteries, or the one may cause the other. A slightly reduced life expectancy (about 2–3 years) is also associated with neuroses in general.

There is a constant presumption, in both popular and more professional literature, that 'stress' can lead to illness such as cancer or strokes. Again, there is very little hard evidence to prove or disprove this, although people who are clinically anxious tend to see the doctor more often. As a result, there is likely to be a bias towards assuming a relationship between being anxious and getting ill, from both the doctor's and the patient's perspectives. However, people who are clinically anxious tend to be more likely to resort to ways of reducing their anxiety by the use of alcohol, drugs, or injurious activities. These will of course bring on their own set of illnesses (especially alcohol dependence), and in that sense anxiety is a genuine aetiological factor.

1.12 Are there really clear signs and symptoms of anxiety?

This is discussed in detail in *Chapter 2*. The essential answer is that symptoms of anxiety are quite typical, tend to have typical cluster patterns, and are not difficult to elicit. Many doctors are fearful of making the diagnosis, a reluctance perhaps based upon an over-acceptance of the objectivity of biochemical tests versus clinical assessment. Remember, the more tests one does the more likelihood there is of obtaining at least one abnormal test result. The rates are something like 5% if there are 5 tests, and up to 20% if there are 20 tests.

1.13 Can one diagnose anxiety confidently and accurately?

Yes – as is outlined in *Chapter 3*, with the processes of diagnosis and differential diagnosis. By and large common things occur commonly, and the pattern of symptoms and the forms of presentation are usually typical. Part of the problem is explaining the nature of the illness to the patient, and choosing the right balance between making a confident diagnosis and doing sensible tests. There are simple series of questions and even specific rating scales (HADS – Hospital and Anxiety Diagnostic Scale – *see Q. 3.2*) which can be used, and these are really quite accurate. As always, taking a good history and carrying out an appropriate examination is the basis of good practice. And *never* tell patients it is all in their mind – anxiety is a most unpleasant physical *and* psychological disorder.

1.14 Why are doctors often so anxious about managing patients with anxiety disorders?

This is usually to do with differing attitudes towards psychological presentations, different levels of training and different levels of interest. It is also true that assessing someone with an anxiety disorder, within the confines of a normal GP appointment time, is really rather difficult. Whether using a clinical method, or a standardized questionnaire, extricating all the details that can confirm the condition can take time.

There is also the problem of transference, which has a technical meaning within psychoanalytic practice, but helps to explain, in a small way, how patients who are anxious can readily make doctors feel anxious. There is the fear of getting the diagnosis wrong, and missing a 'serious' physical illness. There are also the apparently objective and well-defined parameters of physical disorders and biochemical investigations, as opposed to the, possibly subjective, responses required to understand anxiety disorders. Yet the pattern of symptoms is quite clear in the great majority of cases, the very lack of specificity being especially striking.

1.15 What are the causes of anxiety disorders?

These are outlined in *Chapter 4*, and it is clear that genetic, environmental and physical factors all play a part. Generally there is a 'search after meaning' by patients, who want to understand their symptoms and see how they have arisen. As often as not there is no obvious cause, which is why the need for further research in this area could be genuinely helpful in terms of health delivery. Never forget though that what people eat, drink and do routinely during the day are often vital parts of what is making them feel so worried. Muddling cause and effect – is 'stress at work' making someone anxious, or vice versa? – is also very common, but can be hard to explain to some patients. Someone or something to blame, knowing what was the starter event or process, has become a core demand of modern attitudes.

1.16 Are there different types of anxiety disorder?

The short answer is that there certainly are, and this is discussed more fully in the first part of *Chapter 5*. It is generally accepted that there is a spectrum of neurosis, and those with a tendency to anxiety can present, at different times, and at different ages, with different primary problems. Thus people can develop panic symptoms, find it hard to go outdoors – agoraphobia – be socially phobic, or become secondarily depressed. Anxiety can be primarily physical, or can seem to be more part of an obsessional problem or even an over-concern about one's appearance.

In fact the neurosis spectrum, in terms of different diagnoses, has a core basis in terms of enhanced anxiety. The task of trying to sort out these subtypes may seem a touch precious to the frontline GP, but the variable responses to treatment, whether psychological or pharmacological, do seem to show that there are many genuinely different disorders which present with anxiety symptoms. In this

> sense, anxiety can be seen as something like a psychological 'fever', a common denominator for a range of personal or even metabolic (?) problems.

1.17 Are there are any complications with anxiety disorders?

This is discussed in more detail in the second part of *Chapter 5*, but certainly many people with anxiety have superadded problems. These can be due to the effects of the anxiety in itself, the effects of self-treatment for anxiety (e.g. alcohol), or the effects of medical treatments. Most worrying in this regard is when the medical treatment has been inappropriate, for example the use of antimigraine medications for tension headaches. But it is the curse of the condition that anxiety in itself can cause physical problems, and can mask more serious illnesses, in part via the 'crying wolf' dilemma. In social terms, the handicaps of chronic anxiety are legion, whether it be career development, making relationships, or even getting out of the house.

1.18 Are there any drugs that are really effective in anxiety disorders?

Because anxiety disorders tend to be relapsing or chronic, in terms of the patients that visit their GP, there is a general assumption that they are difficult to treat or not worth treating. This is partly because they often go undiagnosed, partly because patients learn to live with their difficulties, and partly because there is a limited understanding of what drugs to use and how. The evidence certainly shows that some medications, from all the different groups of currently available antidepressants, can be extraordinarily effective. Their use is inhibited by the length of time they need to be taken, the tremendous care required in terms of dosage and increasing dosage, the sensitivity to side-effects of anxiety sufferers, and the common problems of non-compliance. The fact is that we do now have effective drug treatments (*see Ch. 6*), and these are not necessarily addictive.

1.19 Can anxiety be treated without using medication?

> While medication certainly is useful, there has been a large research literature over the last 20–30 years, looking at psychological approaches (*see Ch. 7*). These have ranged from simple supportive counselling through to quite sophisticated cognitive behavioural techniques that have been carefully assessed. Helping patients with insight into their problems, and working through the barriers put up by the anxiety symptoms in themselves, are all part of the approach. It is also probably true that a number of alternative therapies are effective in that they do provide the combination of time spent with

the sufferer and the imparting of techniques to reduce symptoms. Learning to relax can be developed in a range of ways, depending on the patient's attributes, culture, age and level of insight.

1.20 What is the usual course of anxiety?

This is considered in more detail in *Chapter 8*, but whether dealing with state anxiety (i.e. anxiety in the face of specific problems or physical disorders) or trait anxiety (i.e. the tendency to be anxious as a 'born worrier'), a relapsing/remitting course is not uncommon. Not unlike certain skin conditions, such as eczema or psoriasis, anxiety sufferers tend to vary in the intensity with which they experience symptoms, and the association with stress is readily (but not always correctly) made. Any treatment approach needs to take this vulnerability on board, in that often enough just knowing that you can be helped, by a sympathetic GP, if things get bad, can in itself reduce the effect of symptoms. The course of the condition does vary, quite considerably, and helping patients establish insight and self-help, over time, can be very rewarding.

1.21 Is anxiety really an illness, or just another way of medicalizing the usual ups and downs of life?

Clinical anxiety – generalized anxiety disorder in the *International Classification of Diseases*, 10th edition (*ICD-10*; WHO 1992) – is a clearly defined condition, and syndromes like panic disorder and social phobia are equally distinctive (*Table 1.2*). Part of the problem of treating anxiety is the reluctance of many patients, especially men, to seek help. Symptoms are attributed to understandable 'stress', to 'a virus', to diet or to social relationships, and many patients might be reluctant to talk about them even with close family members. A sense of personal failure, especially in the workplace – and many working environments try to promote a competitive, 'we can cope', edge – can readily make people feel that they have not lived up to their own or others' expectations.

There is also, usually, no outward and visible sign to define someone as 'ill'. The person who complains of headaches, of not being able to concentrate, of a range of other physical symptoms, or of feeling 'under the weather', is easily reckoned as lacking personal resources, as weak in some way. While this attitude may be more prevalent among men, the increasing similarities between cultural styles of men and women are generating such pressures across the board. The good side of this process, however, is that the acceptance of psychological problems has increased, and many people do have real, treatable, disorders. Being confident in diagnosing and treating these is what this book is about.

TABLE 1.2 *ICD-10* classification of anxiety disorders and related conditions (WHO 1992)*

F40	Phobic anxiety disorders
	.0 Agoraphobia (with/without panic)
	.1 Social phobia
	.2 Specific phobias (e.g. animals, heights)
F41	Other anxiety disorders
	.0 Panic disorder (episodic paroxysmal anxiety)
	.1 Generalized anxiety disorder
	.2 Mixed anxiety/depression
F42	Obsessive–compulsive disorder
F43	Reaction to severe stress
	.0 Acute stress reaction
	.1 Post-traumatic stress disorder
	.2 Adjustment disorders
F44–F48	Dissociative, somatoform (including somatization) and other neurotic disorders, e.g. hypochondriacal, somatoform pain, unspecified

* These are the most important conditions within the categories outlined. The *ICD-10* is based on widespread research and consensus developed by a World Health Organization initiative using numerous field trials. It is expected to require regular revision and updating as experience and diagnostic advances accrue.

1.22 Should GPs be involved in treating the 'worried well'?

Within the field of mental health – ever the Cinderella service – there has increasingly been an emphasis on serious, psychotic illness. The phrase 'the worried well' – or even 'the walking worried' – has emerged, rather cruelly downplaying the difficulties and embarrassments of a large group of people. Yet ignoring this group of patients is most unfair. Malingerers are the exception that proves the rule, as research regularly shows that people visit their doctor because they do have a problem. Behind all those requests for housing transfers, sick notes and disability allowances there is, as often as not, a chronically unwell individual.

Thus while some GPs may prefer to concentrate on 'proper', physical illnesses, it is still perfectly possible for them to be able to recognize anxiety-based conditions so as to point patients in the right direction for treatment. The overlap of physical and psychological symptoms in fact requires the skills of a doctor to clarify what is what, and the GP is best placed for that primary assessment. There is a need for more clinical psychologists and community psychiatric nurses (CPNs), and these are promised in the 2001

NHS Plan (*see Q. 1.23*). But they will have to work in partnership with medical practitioners, and will rely on GPs and psychiatrists to take the vital first step – make the diagnosis.

1.23 What is the best way of getting regular psychiatric input into primary care?

Part of the dilemma for psychiatric services is the government emphasis on severe mental illness, such as schizophrenia and manic depressive disorder, 'risk management' of such conditions, and ensuring continuing support for those patients. This is despite the fact that 90% of what could be called psychiatric consultations take place in primary care, and the great majority of sufferers have anxiety or depressive conditions, such as outlined in this book. The new National Service Framework (NSF) and resulting NHS Plan (as publicized in 2001) have emphasized the importance of access to consultation within primary care, and the proposed employment of extra psychologists to help with just these conditions.

Throughout the country psychiatric liaison clinics have been set up, with varying models used, and usually these are quite successful. Thus patients can be seen by the psychiatrist, or community psychiatric nurse (CPN), in a GP surgery, and direct consultation can take place between GPs and community mental health teams. This provides personal contact, continued education both ways, and ready assessment for all patients, especially the non-psychotic who might feel stigmatized by attending a psychiatric unit. The development of primary care trusts (PCTs) should promote this activity, by building such liaison clinics into the routine contracts they have with mental health trusts. If this sounds like a pious hope, one can only argue that the whole point of having PCTs is to insist on just such resources being made available.

1.24 What will the National Service Framework (NSF) and NHS Plan do for patients with anxiety disorders?

The NSF has set standards in seven different areas of service delivery for mental health, standards which will be regularly assessed. Those relevant to anxiety disorders are listed in *Box 1.1*. Standard 1 concerns mental health promotion, and should encourage anti-discriminatory policies and programmes, making it easier in the long run for patients to be prepared to seek help. Standards 2 and 3 insist on a proper needs assessment and effective treatments (with or without specialist referral) for those with common mental health problems (such as anxiety). Standards 4–7 insist on care planning, hospital resources, carer support and suicide prevention, and thus are less relevant to anxiety management.

The particular resources that should flow from these (especially 2 and 3), include many more primary care psychologists, designed to help with

---

BOX 1.1 Relevant parts of the NSF and NHS Plan

■ Standard 1 – Mental Health Promotion – a lever for the development of education materials and awareness in schools of panic/anxiety states

■ Standard 2 – those with common mental health problems should have needs identified, i.e. a diagnostic and treatment package for anxiety

■ Standard 3 – those with common mental health problems should be offered 'effective treatments', i.e. trained CPNs/psychologists and/or combined 'mood clinics'

■ Standard 6 – a care plan for carers could be most helpful in developing support/intervention skills for *worried* folk

---

providing behavioural and cognitive therapies, and enhanced support for counselling and psychotherapy services that tend, currently, to have long waiting lists.

 PATIENT QUESTIONS

1.25   Am I neurotic or psychotic or what? Will I get schizophrenia or something like that?

Thinking you are silly or going mad is typical of having an anxiety disorder. Terms like 'neurotic' or 'psychotic' are not really very useful, because what the general public means and what the words technically mean are so different. 'Neurosis' describes that group of mental illnesses (like anxiety, depression, obsessions, etc.) that are real conditions but *do not* put you out of touch with reality. By contrast, a psychosis is a severe mental illness (like schizophrenia) that means you cannot think straight and you believe all sorts of things are going on ('delusions') that are not really happening. These meanings are, of course, a long way from the popular (and stigmatizing) views of neurotics as 'weak and useless', and of psychotics as 'mad and dangerous'.

Having a neurosis also means that it would be extremely unusual – rare even – for you to go on to get an illness like schizophrenia. Ways of understanding how these fears arise, and how to deal with them, are part and parcel of this book. The poor understanding of these conditions, by clinicians and lay people alike, is half the problem in their management.

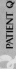 PATIENT QUESTIONS

1.26   Is it possible for a person suffering from panic disorder to have a normal life?

Most people with panic disorder have a 'normal' life, in terms of relationships, work, and getting things done in general. Clearly, those with severe symptoms can be trapped indoors, and feel dominated by their symptoms. But in fact panic disorder, particularly when overlapping with anxiety disorder, is very common, and most people suffering from that probably do not see a doctor, let alone a specialist. This is because the illness tends to come and go, people tend to adapt to it, and many people just insist on getting on with their lives rather than being dominated by their 'nerves'. Even if you do have troubling symptoms, there are many ways of dealing with them, of understanding that you are not going 'mad' or becoming 'a freak', and getting appropriate treatment. It is also possible now to do a range of part-time or specialized jobs that do not involve too much social contact, so that symptoms can be minimized even when you are at work.

Signs and symptoms of anxiety disorders

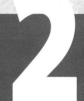

2.1 What are the commonest signs of anxiety?

There are no unequivocal physical signs diagnostic of an anxiety disorder, but this very absence is in itself important. The contrast between the symptoms complained of, over a number of appointments, and the regular lack of physical abnormalities – alongside ever-normal investigations – should alert the GP to the most likely diagnosis. Some patients may have an increased pulse rate, look flushed or frowningly tense, or even show a mild tremor. Some may have non-specific secondary signs, such as bitten nails or nicotine stains, or even a liver edge. Intermittently failed appointments, or only attending with a partner or friend, may indicate that patients have difficulties in getting out on their own. Having a written list of symptoms (do ask if they have one), or repeating questions already dealt with reflects a limited pattern of concentration. A precipitate closure to the consultation may also indicate rising panic.

2.2 What are the commonest symptoms of anxiety?

These are outlined in *Box 2.1*, and are most easily divided into 'head', 'chest', 'GI' (gastrointestinal), 'limbs', and 'mind' complaints. A number of patients present with only one group, while acknowledging some of the others on questioning. Those patients bringing a range of symptoms, physical and psychological, may well find it easier to describe the former than the latter. No one brings a full house, but while almost always stating that they feel 'depressed' or 'worried', anxious folk find it hard to put their finger on what the real problem is. Feeling tired, with or without the rubric 'all the time', feeling generally 'stressed' in some way, or describing a family or work problem, are also typical presentations.

BOX 2.1 Typical complaints of anxious patients

Head
- Confused, light-headed, pressure, headache
- Not real
- Head and neck pain, head tension, funny feeling, feeling sick
- Feeling dizzy
- 'Going to faint'

Chest
- Tightness, heartbeat louder, palpitations
- Chest pain
- Short of breath, breathing too much (hyperventilation), can't catch my breath
- Lump in the throat

BOX 2.1 Typical complaints of anxious patients *(cont'd)*

GI
- Dry mouth
- Pain on and off, wind/bloating, 'butterflies', churning, diarrhoea, feeling sick
- 'A lump'
- Tight/tense

Limbs
- Heavy
- Weakness, sweating (palms), restless
- Jelly legs
- Aching
- Muscle tension, pins and needles
- 'Shaky'
- Unsteady

Psychological/mind
- 'On edge'
- Poor concentration, poor memory, worried
- Feel tired, depressed, irritable, fearful, panics,* 'embarrassed'

* See Box 2.2.

2.3 What is a panic attack?

This describes the sudden onset of an acute sense of panic, often coming on 'out of the blue' with no obvious precipitant. Symptoms are quite disabling, commonly palpitations and dyspnoea with a sense of feeling strange. Feeling dizzy and unsteady are also typical, and patients describe a fear that something awful is going to happen (sense of doom). But, somehow, they do not know what, and this doubles their sense of panic. Fears of doing something silly, of being out of control, of fainting or falling down, or even of dying, are all quite typical. More specific fears, that is of having a heart attack or that they are 'going mad', lead to urgent requests for appointments or A&E attendance. The typical features of a panic attack are outlined in *Box 2.2*. Most patients will have at least five or six of these particular experiences.

Attacks usually last for only a few minutes, but can leave the patient drained and wary for several hours or more. Typically sufferers go outside for fresh air or flee back home. A common result of these attacks – which are a bit like a form of waking epilepsy – is avoidance of places or tasks associated with them, this often being a form of agoraphobia.

> **BOX 2.2 Key features of panic attacks**
> 1. Sudden onset – 'out of the blue'
> 2. Limited duration (minutes rather than hours)
> 3. Overwhelming sense of panic/dislocation
> 4. Distressing physical symptoms
> 5. Irrational fears (of illness/impending doom)
> 6. Urge to flee/go home
> 7. Secondary avoidance of places/circumstances
> 8. Anxiety-prone personality style – 'born worrier'

2.4   What sort of headaches are typical of anxiety?

Headaches are usually of the tension type, tend to be generalized 'all over' the head, and give a feeling of a pressure pushing down. This often extends into the back of the neck and even into the shoulders. Headaches tend to worsen as the day goes on, and despite analgesic use (and abuse) only partially respond to such treatment. Headaches are rarely an isolated symptom. Patients should be asked what other common symptoms they are getting (e.g. muscle tension, tiredness, difficulty getting off to sleep, palpitations). Improvement by using a benzodiazepine is not uncommon, and may therefore even be a diagnostic pointer.

2.5   Do anxious people always somatize?

No. While panic syndrome is by definition associated with a variety of physical symptoms, generalized anxiety disorder (GAD) is often just a sense of feeling worried. Symptoms such as restlessness, feeling uncertain and feeling tired are non-specific and may not be described as physical. Psychological symptoms, such as poor concentration, intrusive ruminations, or lack of self-confidence, are more readily described by better educated, more 'intelligent' patients, but not necessarily so. Nor does such symptomatology always mean better insight. However, given that these presentations are often less severe than when physical symptoms prevail, they should therefore respond more readily to simple psychological treatments.

2.6   Can physical symptoms occur without any obvious feeling of 'anxiety'?

Yes. Many patients see themselves as only having a specific 'disorder', for example asthma, and will focus entirely on the physical symptoms. They may agree, on questioning, to other physical symptoms, but can be indignant when 'worries' or 'anxiety' are mooted. This may be quite genuine, in that they do not experience a sense of fear or anxiety, or due to denial (especially in men) generated by stigma. Such presentations virtually force the GP into a physical/investigative approach, but over time other symptoms or problems will usually emerge, helping to clarify the diagnosis. Check back in the notes; they can be very illuminating.

The various physical symptoms commonly occurring in anxiety are shown in *Figure 2.1*.

2.7 Can one confidently separate out anxiety-based chest symptoms, such as palpitations or chest pain?

Although difficult in some patients, most of the time this is perfectly possible to achieve, assuming the GP knows the patient. Anxiety disorders are usually apparent by one's 20s, and will be reflected in terms of previous notes and attendances. Episodic chest symptoms, coming on alongside feelings of panic or anxiety in younger (i.e. under 30-year-old) patients are much easier to distinguish. They will not be precipitated by physical effort, and there will be lots of positives on asking about other symptoms, such as those outlined in *Box 2.1*.

The safety bias, towards assuming there is a cardiac disease until disproven, is simply out of date if a clear and corroborated history is taken. Patients of course may insist on an ECG, chest X-ray, blood tests etc. – and do not always refuse to do these – but starting off by telling them that anxiety is the most likely diagnosis and what is the necessary treatment (while agreeing it is a physical disease) can be most useful in the long term.

2.8 Do people with established heart disease have different symptoms when anxious?

No one knows the answer to this. Older patients may easily develop an agitated depression, which will present with palpitations and poor sleep, and even episodes of breathlessness. By and large, phlegmatic souls do not get such symptoms, but 'born worriers' will show evidence of worrying throughout their notes. Symptoms will not distinguish true heart disease from anxiety or panic disorder, but signs will. The combination of signlessness (i.e. no oedema, cyanosis, raised JVP) with variable and/or multiple symptomatology is a sure indication that this is not – or highly unlikely to be – primary heart disease.

2.9 Do anxious patients often complain of pins and needles, and is there any particular pattern to this?

Pins and needles, in the hands or even the face, are typical complaints of those who hyperventilate. By blowing off their CO_2 they develop a relative hypocapnia, that is to say a low blood CO_2. This alters their acid–base

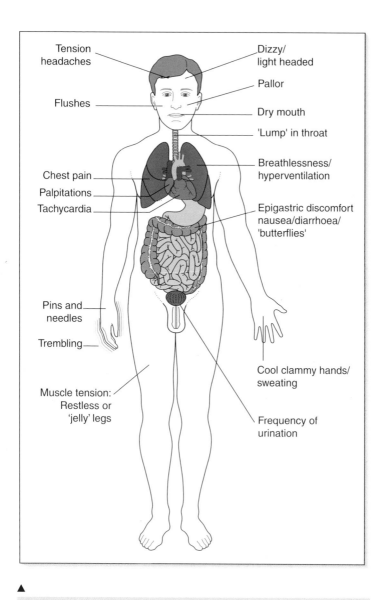

Fig. 2.1 Somatic clinical features of generalized anxiety disorder. (After Puri et al 1996)

balance, affects calcium levels and creates the symptoms of paraesthesia, (i.e. pins and needles). Such experiences are almost always episodic, associated with feeling tense and/or panicky, and reinforce feelings of a serious physical disorder, for example 'a stroke' or 'multiple sclerosis'. The symptoms can often be reproduced in the surgery by getting the patient to breathe in and out very quickly.

2.10 Is the common complaint of feeling 'tired all the time' (TATT) often a symptom of anxiety?

Yes. Tiredness occurs since people do not sleep well, and report subjective daytime tiredness. This may represent poor concentration, feeling muddled and feeling not right, as much as true fatigue. They can also find tranquillizers helpful. Differentiating between anxiety tiredness and other causes, such as depression or anaemia, needs of course a careful outlining of associated symptoms. Tired all the time folk, who are primarily anxious, will have a nice selection of other symptoms, across a range of bodily areas. They are also, often, physically unfit via the vicious circle of anxiety, insomnia, feeling drained, not doing much but worrying about it.

2.11 Is there a particular pattern of symptoms, or do they vary a lot?

There is a typical pattern – for panic attacks especially – and the standard set of questions should quickly elicit what is going on. A selection from *Box 2.1* is particularly helpful. Patients may vary in the dominant area of symptomatology, for example the head rather than the abdomen, but the very number of symptoms (usually half a dozen at least), the daytime limitations for example on travel, and a common avoidance of social or crowded situations will be there. The more symptoms the clearer the diagnosis, especially if they involve a number of different organ groups.

2.12 Do sufferers often exaggerate their symptoms?

This may seem so, but most people do not in fact like being ill. It is partly a cultural phenomenon as to how we learn to present ourselves to doctors, and stiff upper lip English phlegmatism is not as typical as it seems to have been in the past. Studies on malingering or even 'hysterical' behaviours regularly show that most of the subjects do have real symptoms, do not try to fool their doctors, and do not like being unwell. Of course, there are always exceptions to the rule, especially when disability allowances are on the line. It is also worth realizing that the typical pattern of symptoms is quite difficult to make up, and throwing in a few irrelevant queries (such as 'do you see strange colours?' or 'do you dream about snakes a lot?') can help clarify matters quickly. Most patients, though, will simply look puzzled at these suggestions.

2.13 Do patients with clinical anxiety sometimes present looking quite unworried?

This is a typical presentation. There are no hard and fast signs of clinical anxiety, and putting on a good face is reinforced by the stigma of mental illness. It is only by clarifying details of patients' concerns, even asking them to make a list of their problems in order of severity for example, that a diagnostic pattern can emerge. In this sense the classic old presentation of hysteria, called 'la belle indifférence' (best translated as 'the mask of tranquillity'), is representative of the ready tendency we all have, consciously or unconsciously, to cover up (or try to cover up) internal anxiety.

2.14 Do anxious patients often complain of depression?

This is probably their commonest complaint and the commonest form of presentation. Because the difficulties generated by anxiety create a sense of things not being quite right, people naturally feel 'depressed' at what is happening. They also may well have one or two other more obviously depressive symptoms, but tend to gloss over what is actually making them feel depressed. It is always worth asking how depression affects an individual, whether it makes the person feel low/slow/tired or edgy/anxious/tense? Many patients would agree on the latter, and an anxiety disorder will emerge.

It is not surprising therefore that a pattern of constantly failed antidepressant therapy can be seen in patients' notes. Not having been diagnosed properly, and being readily intolerant of side-effects, they keep stopping them but keep coming back because of their concerns. Of course mixed anxiety/depression does exist (at least officially – *see Box 2.3*) but clarifying one way or the other is well worth the effort in terms of treatment approaches. There are, nevertheless, a number of overlapping symptoms between anxiety and depression, and the relationship is portrayed in *Figure 2.2*.

BOX 2.3 Mixed anxiety and depression disorder (*ICD-10* category F41.2)

- ■ Anxiety *and* depressive symptoms present
- ■ Both sets of symptoms are *mild*
- ■ Just *worry* and/or *over-concern* is not diagnostic
- ■ If due to recent stressor (e.g. bereavement) consider an *adjustment disorder*
- ■ Most 'cases' never come to medical attention

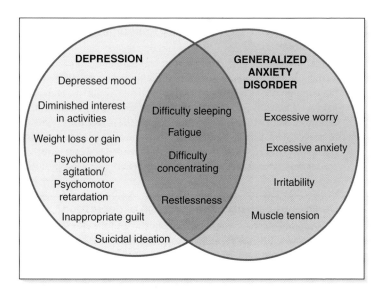

▲

Fig. 2.2 Depression and GAD have specific overlapping symptoms.

2.15 Do anxious patients tend to have any particular effect on you, the clinician?

The way a patient affects a doctor is regarded as a key part of making a diagnosis in psychiatric training. Doctors vary in their temperament and levels of patience, with certain reactions being very common. For example, anxious patients often have an aura of urgency, with pressure put upon the GP to *do* something now. Feeling pushed or irritable because of this should help with the diagnosis. Alternatively, having a sense that a patient does not feel confident, or wants a second – or even a third – opinion, is also quite common. These reactions can be extraordinarily useful, in that they reflect in part what psychoanalysts call 'the transference'. Such an approach does mean that doctors have to ask themselves, as a normal routine, how consultations make them feel.

2.16 Is feeling dizzy a particular symptom?

Yes. This is very common indeed, reflecting the sense of light-headedness and feeling unsteady on one's legs that constantly occurs in anxiety and/or panic states. People often complain of dizzy spells, and need to be pushed to explain this. What do they in fact mean by 'dizzy'? Do they, for example, think they will faint, or feel confused? – and in what circumstances does this happen? Like the term 'depression', feeling 'dizzy' tends to be used as a broad-church, overall description covering a wide range of symptoms. Never accept such language at face value, and use the hyperventilation challenge to see if that reproduces the symptoms.

2.17 Are eye or eyesight problems often due to anxiety?

People readily complain of blurred vision or eye pain, of a non-specific nature, in the context of anxiety states. However, this is not a common presentation, and anxiety should be a bit further back in the differential diagnosis. There is certainly a group of patients who wear tinted glasses, seem sensitive to light, and worry constantly about their eyes, but these are usually distinct. New, specific visual problems should be carefully checked, especially if patients are already on antidepressants, because tricyclics especially affect one's ability to focus. Again, if there is a wider pattern of symptoms, involving other parts of the body as well as the eyes, then anxiety does become much more likely as the core diagnosis.

2.18 Are weight and appetite loss typical of clinical anxiety?

No. These symptoms are typically depressive, and should bias one to assuming that that is the diagnosis, unless there are other obvious physical problems. Many anxious patients complain of picking at their food, because of tension, but do not seem to lose significant (i.e. more than half a stone) amounts of weight. Comfort-eating is a much more likely problem, while overtly anxious people who are shaking and trembling – and displaying obvious weight loss – should make one think at once about alcohol or drug dependence, or even a thyroid problem.

2.19 Is feeling sick or nauseated a typical symptom?

Feeling 'sick with tension' is very common, although patients do not commonly vomit in public. A stressful ordeal, like attending court or making a presentation, is a typical precipitant. Again this is usually part of a pattern of symptoms (*see Box 2.1*), particularly when gastrointestinal concerns predominate. If this is the only symptom, then one has a dilemma. Clarifying the circumstances, for example, do they only feel sick when in public, can be of help. Nausea and 'butterflies' in the stomach when faced with social contacts are common symptoms of social phobia.

2.20 Do anxious patients actually fall down and faint or do they just complain of feeling faint?

It is most unusual for anxiety to make a patient actually fall down. The absence of falls and faints, despite the complaints, should alert one to the diagnosis. Anxious patients regularly feel 'as if' they will collapse, fall, lose control, etc., and they may have to sit down and put their head between their knees to recover, but they do not actually lose consciousness. The contrast between the awful way they feel, i.e. unwell and unsteady, and what happens to them, is again often quite striking. Dramatic, apparent respiratory arrests – sometimes with odd posturing and arms held stiff – are unusual but well-recognized phenomena in the very anxious. Though rather alarming, especially to relatives or lay folk, they are helpfully diagnostic.

2.21 How common is feeling unsteady, or feeling your legs are like jelly, as a symptom of anxiety?

This is an absolutely classic symptom. Almost all patients with panic disorder describe this, or something akin to it. It is a combination of light-headedness, often due to hyperventilation, and (probably) a central impairment of balance. It wears off as the panic wears off, but is a key factor in generating avoidance of places because of a natural fear of embarrassment, or falling or fainting in public. An alternative description is a sense that the ground does not seem to be firm or even seems to be wobbly. And, of course, despite this strange sensation, patients hardly ever fall down.

2.22 Does anxiety have any particular nose or mouth symptoms?

There are no common symptoms affecting the nose, but a dry mouth is quite typical. Patients lick their lips, feel dry, feel hoarse, and even find it hard to speak clearly. The sense of something being caught in the throat, like a lump (so-called 'globus hystericus'), is also well known. Such mouth symptoms, although typical for generalized anxiety, are especially so in social phobia, worsening the fear of speaking in public for example. Idiosyncratic patterns of behaviour can make people scratch their nose or bite their lips when tense, but this is more of a behavioural sign than what the patient will complain of.

2.23 Is a resting tremor typical in anxiety, or is there any other particular form of movement disorder associated with it?

Tremor is not as common as one would think. It certainly can occur, and this may be a family or long-standing personal trait. A tremor of recent onset should make one worry about alcohol dependence, or withdrawal, or even thyrotoxicosis. There are no other obvious movement disorder presentations, but all patients with an established tic or movement syndrome (e.g. chorea) show enhanced movement when feeling more anxious. Likewise, psychiatric patients with pre-existing dyskinesia, usually secondary to dopamine-blocking medication, are always much more shaky and twitchy when they are feeling anxious or tense. It is always worth just watching patients – rather than listening to them – for half a minute or so, to check on their degree and type of movement. Early-onset chorea, or other dyskinesias, often get completely missed or dismissed as understandable restlessness.

 PATIENT QUESTIONS

2.24   Why do I feel so strange and scared?

Anxiety and panic attacks tend to fool you – or rather your brain – into thinking that something dreadful is going to happen. It is meant to be an alarm system, disturbing enough to protect you from danger and get you into the 'fight or flight' response. It is not surprising therefore that panicking men often turn angry and lash out, while women run away to safety (i.e. home). The 'strange' feeling is called 'depersonalization', because people feel unreal and cut off from the world. Being 'scared' is the effect of too much adrenaline washing through you, making you sweat, breathe faster, tremble, etc. – even making your hair prick up on the back of your neck (when we were primitive ape men this helped let off the heat from our overactive, hairy, bodies). The way you feel is real; but just like a flurry of rain, it will pass quite quickly.

2.25   Why do I tremble and why do my hands shake when I am feeling anxious?

This is one of the most common symptoms of anxiety, although many people have what is called an 'essential' tremor, for no obvious reason. This will come and go depending on the situation they find themselves in. Tremors and shakes are essentially to do with increased muscle tension. Perhaps the most vivid image of this is when a weightlifter is straining to keep a heavy dumb-bell over his head, and as he strains and concentrates, his legs or trunk or arms start to shake a bit, or quite a lot, particularly if he is about to drop the weight. The increased adrenaline pumping through your system overheats the natural mechanism, the strained muscles keep contracting strongly, but not in balance, and tremor emerges. The good thing about having a tremor or trembles is that it is a strong sign, when it comes and goes in anxious situations, that you do suffer from anxiety. Some forms of medication, however, can cause a shake, and a tremor at rest (when you are not straining at anything or embarrassed or trying to do something in public) that has come on in later life is always worth checking out with your doctor.

Diagnosing anxiety and the differential diagnosis

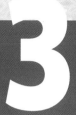

DIFFERENTIATING PSYCHOSES SUCH AS SCHIZOPHRENIA

3.1 Is it really possible to make a diagnosis of anxiety in the few minutes of a GP consultation?

The simple answer is yes. The only assumption made by this is that the patient is known to the GP; thus the personality, background and history of previous presentations is available in the notes. Bearing this in mind, and eliciting the pattern of symptoms that people commonly have, alongside no evidence of any significant physical disorder, in terms of examination or investigations, makes for a positive diagnosis. Anxiety should *not* be a diagnosis of exclusion, because that can turn into a complex, repetitive (and often confrontational) bottomless pit. The core features of the symptoms, and especially the presence of panic episodes, are as reliable as any 'physical' sign. Confirmation from a (*sensible*) partner or family member will often clinch matters.

3.2 Are there any useful diagnostic rating scales?

Yes. Although a number have been published, the most practical and effective is called the 'Hospital Anxiety and Depression Scale' (HADS), first published in 1983 (*Fig. A1.1, p. 145*). It is very simple to fill in, is filled in by the patients themselves, and takes only several minutes to complete. Patients should be told not to think too hard about questions, but, literally, to state how they felt over the last week or so. Immediate, gut reactions are much more important in this questionnaire, in terms of its validity, than people sitting and thinking about it for a long time.

It is generally accepted that a score of less than 8 is normal, while over 10 is clinically significant. It can also be used, of course, to assess how patients feel sequentially, and thus help them look at their response to treatment, time or whatever. There are a number of other scales, either self-rating or clinician administered (e.g. the Impact of Event Scale (*Fig. A1.2, p. 146*), measuring the degree of subjective post-traumatic stress – *see also Q. 5.18*), but none is any better in terms of reliability or validity than any other. The important thing is to use one regularly, so as to get a good clinical feel for it.

3.3 Are there any background questions that are particularly useful in establishing the diagnosis?

The most useful approach for the clinician, and it is time well spent, is to check the background notes. Frequency of attendance, the range of symptoms (*Fig. 3.1*), use of a range of antidepressants, anxiolytics or even analgesic medications, and previous investigations (essentially negative) are all characteristic. In terms of direct questions, a simple one like 'Are you

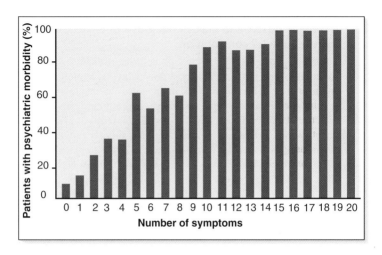

▲

Fig. 3.1 Association between number of unexplained physical symptoms and psychiatric disorder (anxiety and depression) in an international study of primary care attenders. (From Mayou & Farmer 2002, with permission of the BMJ Publishing Group.)

something of a born worrier?', or 'Do you tend to check things regularly?', are useful. Questions about whether patients like things to be very neat and tidy (to give an idea of obsessional traits), or whether they ever find it hard to leave the house, are also useful. A corroborative history is vital, and a friend or relative should be invited to come along, if necessary, on another appointment. Getting the patient to go through a typical day, in terms of sleeping, getting up, doing things, going out, eating, meeting people etc., can be most revealing.

3.4 How can one differentiate between generalized anxiety disorder (GAD) and panic attacks?

Although these two conditions regularly overlap, and should be best seen as part of a spectrum of enhanced anxiety, the key difference is the presence or not of panic attacks. Generalized anxiety is characterized by the constant tendency to worry about things, leading to a degree of restlessness and difficulty getting off to sleep. Even the most trivial concern causes worry, which impairs concentration and even recall, and makes patients wary and depressed at their constant state of psychological discomfort. This background may not be so obvious in panic syndrome, although commonly there will be similar symptoms prior to the first panic attack. Panic attacks (*see Box 2.2*) are typical in their sudden onset, the severe combination of physical and psychological symptoms, their natural resolution over the course of 10 minutes or so, and the resultant avoidance they create.

3.5 Is it really possible to distinguish between anxiety and depression?

Yes, about half the time. That is to say, many anxious patients complain of accompanying depressive symptoms, and vice versa. There is a big overlap in some of these symptoms, for example feeling tired by day, difficulty sleeping, impaired concentration and feeling generally 'not right', but people can generally say what their dominant mood is. That is to say, do they generally feel tense, worried, unable to relax, or do they feel slow, low and negative? Again, it is most important to ask what they mean by the term 'depressed' or 'worried', and to try to elicit specific symptoms. Despite all this, a number of people do seem to have a mixed anxiety/depression picture (*Box 2.3*) and then treatment (*see Chs 6 and 7*) will depend on the specific symptoms. Again, use of a specific rating scale (*see Q. 3.2*) can be helpful.

3.6 Can patients be anxious and depressed at the same time?

Essentially yes. The prevalence of mixed anxiety and depression shows the limits of our current diagnostic understanding of these conditions, in that they remain syndromes rather than tight diagnoses. The term 'cothymia' has even been suggested as a specific, mixed picture, diagnosis (*see Box 8.1*). Nevertheless, it is very common for patients to complain of depression as a secondary response to their anxiety and even panic attacks, without mentioning the fact that they cannot go outdoors (unless particularly asked about it). Furthermore, patients will often talk about being anxious or depressed because of something else, whether it be a bereavement, another physical symptom, or a social problem. If no clear pattern emerges it is still possible to organize an appropriate treatment programme, taking things symptom by symptom.

3.7 Do anxious patients commonly have a raised blood pressure or pulse rate?

No. They may well complain of feeling their heart beat loudly, or of headaches that they feel are due to 'blood pressure', but parameters are by and large normal. Even a patient feeling quite intensely embarrassed and anxious, perhaps due to social phobia, will often have no obvious pulse or BP problem. Checking these can be most useful, however, so as to reassure patients and to let them know that you do understand that their problem may have a physical component.

3.8 What are the most important investigations that can eliminate physical illness?

If the patient is not well known to you, then it is worth doing a basic screen if there are marked symptoms of enhanced physical and psychological arousal. Whether these are based around chest symptoms, or head symptoms, or a mixture of everything, it is always worth checking on full blood count and ESR (especially if the patient may have come from abroad with some rare disease), and doing liver function tests with measurement of gamma-glutamyl transferase (gamma-GT) (looking for abnormality secondary to alcohol). If there are obvious clinical indications, then thyroid function tests should be carried out (but *not* routinely), while an ECG and chest X-ray are always worth doing in people who smoke, are overweight, or who ask directly for them. Any more complex investigations are not worth doing, unless there are highly specific clinical indicators, and even then they should probably be left to hospital specialists. A particularly useless investigation is a skull X-ray, unless of course there is a clear history of a head injury or clear, new, visual impairments.

3.9 Can one clinically separate out anxiety and thyrotoxicosis?

Not always, but usually. The basic difference is in the resting pulse, if you can persuade a partner to feel the pulse when the patient is asleep at night. Thyrotoxics will have a continually raised pulse, day and night, not just in the 'stress' of the surgery. Likewise they will be weather sensitive (feeling sweaty in hotter weather and preferring the cooler weather), often have a small goitre and/or eye signs, and will have a pattern of a new onset of symptoms. By contrast the anxious are anxious in all weathers, possibly feeling worse in winter when they feel 'depressed', will have no obvious eye or neck signs, and will have a constant pattern of feeling worried. Though having a wider range of symptoms, they will not, for example, have lost weight.

3.10 Is anaemia, of any form, an important differential diagnosis for anxiety?

Probably yes, because the tiredness associated with iron deficiency anaemia can overlap readily with that of people who describe feeling 'tired all the time'. A pattern of heavy periods, or poor diet, can compound this. Abnormalities in the mean corpuscular volume (MCV) (it is raised in many people with alcohol dependence syndrome) will also lead to your pathology laboratory querying a macrocytic anaemia. In this sense, the macrocytosis, as a marker for alcohol, becomes a secondary marker for the anxiety generating the alcohol abuse. There is no other association of a formal anaemia with clinical anxiety states, although iron deficiency is associated with restless legs at night (so-called Ekbom's syndrome).

3.11 Should one routinely do an ECG (electrocardiogram) on anxious patients?

This should not be a routine, if the pattern of symptoms (*see Q. 2.2*) is quite typical. If there is a clear focus on episodic palpitation, and the history of panic episodes is not quite as clear as one would like, then a routine ECG is helpful, can be reassuring for the patient (sometimes!), and is a safe option. As always, it is worth advising the patient that it is merely to reassure you, that you expect it to be normal, and that it is a very simple examination.

3.12 Can an EEG (electroencephalogram) be helpful in excluding neurological causes of anxiety?

An EEG has a very limited place in the diagnosis of anxiety disorders. There is no evidence of any significant abnormality in those suffering from anxiety or panic syndromes, and no specific pattern or reactivity even slightly associated with such states. Even if the differential diagnosis is between panic attacks and some form of epilepsy, for example temporal lobe epilepsy (TLE), then again the EEG may not be helpful. The clinical pattern of seizures as described by the patient is the basis for a firm diagnosis of epilepsy, which *cannot* be excluded by a 'normal' EEG. Non-specific abnormalities in the EEG are of course noted in space-occupying lesions, but unless there are specific clinical indicators (e.g. memory loss, neurological signs), an EEG is not usually indicated.

3.13 What are the indications for carrying out a brain CT or MRI scan?

In patients presenting with anxiety disorders, a CT or MRI scan is unlikely to be helpful, unless there are specific clinical indicators. These will include neurological signs of a possible intracerebral lesion, for example cranial nerve abnormalities or an abnormal optic fundus. In terms of the mental state examination, only clear evidence of cognitive impairment, such as disorientation or significant memory loss, would be an indication for radiological investigations. While non-specific anxiety may be a presenting symptom for some space-occupying lesions, the clinical picture is usually one of perplexity and slowing down rather than agitation and over-arousal.

3.14 Should one routinely screen for illicit drugs, such as amfetamines, cocaine or ecstasy?

Abnormal anxiety states, with or without episodes of panic, particularly when accompanied by perceptual abnormalities (for example hallucinations) or patients being distressed by feeling 'weird' or very depersonalized, are common accompaniments of some forms of drug use. Symptoms may be a direct result of ingesting illicit drugs, particularly the unreliable cocktails handed out under the rubric of 'E' (ecstasy). Likewise, withdrawal states from drug usage, in the immediate aftermath, or after prolonged tranquillizer, opiate or even cannabis dependence – as well as from some antidepressants – tend to mimic anxiety disorders. A low threshold to carrying out a routine drug screen, particularly when younger patients are involved, is very sensible and the test is easily done. Most hospital laboratories do a routine screen, requiring only a single urine sample, covering the standard range of drugs of abuse. The hospital pathologist may have to be contacted, however, as to the sensitivity of the assay performed, and certain drugs (e.g. cocaine) are eliminated very quickly (within 48 hours) and thus are more difficult to detect.

It is probably best to be quite open with patients when suggesting a drug screen, not least because their reaction to such a proposal may in itself be quite informative. Illicit drug use and/or abuse is so common now that a substantial diagnosis often cannot be reached unless this aspect has been clarified.

3.15 Are there any useful tests for alcohol dependence?

The most useful test for alcohol dependence is the CAGE questionnaire. This is summarized in *Box 3.1*, and consists of four questions related to alcohol usage. The important clinical point is to ask patients a first question, 'Have you Cut down alcohol recently?' *before* asking the question as to how much the patient might be drinking. One positive answer means that alcohol abuse is probable, while two makes it almost certain. The features of alcohol dependence are summarized in *Box 3.2*.

In terms of blood tests, the mean corpuscular volume (MCV) is raised in between one-half and two-thirds of those with alcohol problems, while the gamma-glutamyl transferase (gamma-GT) is raised in about 70–80%. Again, however, these tests are not exclusive, some 20%, or even more, of alcoholics showing no haematological or biochemical abnormality whatsoever. In this sense the CAGE questionnaire is probably more sensitive than the MCV or gamma-GT values, picking up some 90% of patients.

> **BOX 3.1 The CAGE questionnaire for alcohol dependence**
> 1. Have you ever felt you should **C**ut down, or have you recently **C**ut down, on your drinking?
> 2. Have you ever felt **A**nnoyed, or got into arguments, because of your drinking or people's comments about it?
> 3. Have you ever felt bad or **G**uilty about your drinking?
> 4. Have you needed an **E**ye-opener, for any reason at all (i.e. a drink first thing in the morning on waking)?
>
> NB: An alcoholic's first drink might be at midday or even later, the individual having only woken shortly before that.

> **BOX 3.2 Features of the alcohol dependence syndrome**
> - Narrowing of the drinking repertoire
> - Salience (prioritization) of drinking
> - Increased tolerance to alcohol
> - Repeated withdrawal symptoms
> - Relief or avoidance of withdrawal symptoms by further drinking
> - Subjective awareness of a compulsion to drink
> - Reinstatement of drinking after abstinence

3.16 Is anxiety sometimes due to excessive caffeine intake?

Yes. The prevalence of this is hard to gauge, but caffeinism, namely being somewhat aroused, edgy, sweaty and having an increased pulse rate, can certainly be generated by excessive coffee or tea drinking. Half a dozen cups of relatively strong black coffee a day can lead to such symptoms, depending on the patient's sensitivity, the symptoms worsening with additional cups. Likewise with tea, more than about 10 cups a day could lead to caffeinist effects, and high intakes of diet drinks and/or chocolate may also produce symptoms. A routine question in the assessment of anxious patients is some sort of quantification of their caffeine (essentially tea and coffee) intake, because sometimes intakes can be quite extraordinary (i.e. 20 or 30 cups a day).

3.17 Is it common to confuse a panic attack with a heart attack?

This is a very typical problem, not least because of the degree of conviction of certain patients that they are having a heart attack, when they are having a panic attack. Not uncommonly they may have been sensitized to heart problems by cardiac illness running in the family, or by a friend or family member having recently suffered a genuine heart attack. Differentiating between the symptoms can be difficult, but a positive diagnosis can be made with a clear history. Thus, panic attacks occur out of the blue, with no relationship to exertion, and generate a wide range of symptoms both physical and psychological. They are commoner in women, include a sense of panic or depersonalization, and resolve after a few minutes. By contrast, cardiac events are much more likely to be related to exertion, have symptoms essentially confined to the chest or upper abdomen, occur anywhere (not just in the crowded places associated with panics) and are more likely in older males. They do not resolve in 5 or 10 minutes.

3.18 How can one differentiate a panic attack from an acute asthmatic episode?

Again this is difficult in someone with a known history of asthma, and particularly when patients find it hard to describe their symptoms. Classically asthmatics find it hard to breathe out, while those who are suffering from a panic attack describe difficulty getting air in. They will not have an audible wheeze, will complain of some sort of throat constriction, and will often have a range of other symptoms (e.g. palpitations, depersonalization, jelly legs). Oddly enough a history of inhaler use, while probably indicative of genuine asthma, may not necessarily be diagnostic, and of course beta stimulants can enhance anxiety.

DIFFERENTIATING PSYCHOSES SUCH AS SCHIZOPHRENIA

3.19 Can anxiety be the presentation of a more serious mental illness such as schizophrenia?

It is very typical for patients with schizophrenia to present with a non-specific form of anxiety. This may be a state of inarticulate perplexity, part of what is called a 'delusional mood'. Patients will describe a sense of something going on but they are not quite sure what, a state of uncertainty about themselves, and a sense of having changed. Some will describe ideas of reference, that is a belief that people are looking at them or even following them around. This enhanced self-consciousness is sometimes difficult to distinguish from the way agoraphobic patients feel when they are in a state of panic.

In general schizophrenic patients, especially those suffering from a paranoid form of schizophrenia, will describe specific incidents, and the sense that this is *really* happening, for example people *are* laughing at them.

By contrast, anxious patients will describe an 'as if' sense of people looking at them, knowing the thought to be silly but finding it hard to put it out of their mind. An anxiety or depressive disorder, particularly with diffuse symptoms, may be the prodrome to a more serious psychotic illness, but again there will usually be specific symptoms (e.g. of perplexity or odd beliefs) mixed in with the more non-specific anxiety.

3.20 Does clinical anxiety often go on to present as a paranoid state?

No. While paranoid symptoms, that is to say the belief that one is in a special relationship to what is going on around one (the coincidental becomes significant) can mimic anxious self-consciousness, the great majority of anxious patients do not develop formal paranoid delusions. They may feel rather self-conscious in public places, especially when panicking, and may worry that they are becoming paranoid, or even use the term 'paranoid'. If asked, however, they will almost always agree that they do not really believe they are being followed, threatened, or whatever, but they just find it hard to put the idea out of their mind that someone is looking at them or 'taking the mickey'. The combination of enhanced anxiety and paranoid ideas is very common in people with alcohol problems, especially when withdrawing, and this flavour of presentation should therefore lead to a close consideration of the patient's alcohol usage. Most clinical anxiety simply goes on as clinical anxiety, unless progressing to formal panic attacks as well.

3.21 Are patients with schizophrenia or manic depressive psychosis often troubled by anxiety symptoms as well?

Such patients usually do not have formal panic attacks, but a prodromal non-specific anxiety is not uncommon prior to the onset of any form of psychosis. Patients with insight will be particularly affected, noting for example a change in sleep pattern and mood state (in the case of manic depressives). Patients with an established diagnosis therefore, of for example a schizophrenic illness, and developing symptoms, should be carefully assessed because of the likelihood of a more serious relapse. In terms of general management, especially for patients with schizophrenia, reducing the atmosphere of emotional expression in their families is a key factor in relapse prevention. Increasing anxiety can therefore be used as a warning sign for more active treatment, and should be built in to the management approach for such patients.

3.22 Can some physical disorders in themselves cause a formal anxiety disorder?

There is currently no evidence for this, although research into the aetiology of anxiety and panic attacks certainly points to abnormalities of brain biochemical activity. Enhanced levels of arousal may be caused by a stroke or other form of brain damage, and anxiety symptoms are very prominent in post-traumatic stress disorder (PTSD) as well as some post-concussional syndromes. The investigations for anxiety disorders (*see Q. 3.8*) are of course an important facet of diagnosis and management. Treatment of such underlying disorders should by definition eliminate the secondary anxiety symptoms.

3.23 Is there any significance in the wearing of dark glasses, or having many tattoos, ear/nose rings?

While tattoos and infibulation are now a much more acceptable aspect of modern life, there is no evidence that they have any specific association with anxiety, panic, or even depressive disorders. Likewise the fashionable wearing of dark glasses, although sometimes seen by certain physicians as a sign of 'neuroticism' or even hypochondria, is not especially diagnostic. However, the alerting effect of drugs such as amfetamines or cocaine may make some people more light sensitive, and there certainly is a tendency among some chronic users to wear 'shades', for practical as well as style reasons. If anything, the natural tendency of people suffering from anxiety or panic disorders is to *not* stand out in a crowd, so anonymous clothing and limited self-decoration is probably much more likely.

3.24 What about patients who use a written list of symptoms?

The use of a written list of symptoms may be deemed sensible, obsessional, annoying, or as somehow diagnostic. However, while the presentation of a 'little list' (la maladie des petits points) probably represents nothing more or less than a certain obsessionality, for some patients it is quite a sensible precaution. Anxious folk tend to find it hard to concentrate, to worry about forgetting and thus more readily to forget, and to feel concerned that they have not given out the full details of their illness. Such little lists can in fact be extremely helpful in quickly reaching a diagnosis, since they will outline a range of symptoms (typical in anxiety) (*Fig. 3.1*), can be a useful basis for discussion, and can even help shorten the consultation. Welcoming such approaches, or even suggesting to patients who find it hard to clarify their symptoms that they come back at a later date having put a list together (perhaps along with their partner) may be a key part of the therapeutic relationship.

3.25 Does anxiety cause any sexual problems?

Formal anxiety disorders can interfere with all aspects of sexual relationships, from the simple process of meeting people to more intimate details of sexual performance. Patients with social phobia are particularly prone to feeling 'foolish', having a dry mouth and finding it hard to articulate when confronted with the daunting problem of taking someone out. Likewise patients will feel rather foolish at having to explain their symptoms, because of the usual accompaniments of stigma, misunderstanding and impaired concentration.

In terms of common, practical sexual problems, anorgasmia in females and premature ejaculation in males are likely to be enhanced by states of anxiety. Formal referral to a qualified sex therapist, to help with techniques for self-relaxation, can be a most effective approach to such difficulties. However, there is no evidence that clinical anxiety is in itself the cause of such sexual problems, given their general level of prevalence in the population.

3.26 Can severe anxiety cause symptoms like hallucinations?

An hallucination is a perception in the absence of a stimulus, for example seeing or hearing something when there is actually nothing there. This needs to be distinguished from an illusion or misinterpretation, whereby a real image may be misinterpreted because of anxiety or confusion. Thus anxious people may worry that footsteps behind them represent a possible threat, or when walking along a dark country lane may over-interpret the meaning of something rustling in the bushes. This, however, is not a true hallucination, even though a number of people tend to use the term to describe a range of unusual visual phenomena, when they are tired, have taken drugs, or when they are half-asleep/half-awake in the middle of the night.

A number of patients, however, do have what is called a pseudo-hallucination, that is a sense of a voice inside their head, telling them things or even telling them to do things. Such a symptom is not specifically associated with anxiety or panic states, and needs to be carefully explored. Of course, if patients are genuinely hallucinating, for example convinced that the neighbours next door are spying on them and making rude comments about them, then it is likely that the anxiety is part and parcel of the early symptoms of a psychotic illness like schizophrenia.

3.27 Can anxiety make a patient genuinely forgetful?

Yes. Concern about forgetfulness or 'losing one's mind' is a very typical symptom of patients with anxiety, not least because they sometimes find it hard to register information. This is related to impaired concentration, since they are focusing perhaps on their anxiety symptoms, for example why is their heart beating so fast? Because of this state of distraction they cannot recall clearly what has been happening, and feel they have therefore 'forgotten' something. When flustered they often tend to lose things, and this enhances further their sense of forgetfulness, their fear that maybe they have a serious brain illness, and their anxiety about their other symptoms. Some patients can be quickly reassured by getting them to answer some simple questions about recent events, for example what they saw on television the night before, or what has recently been in the news. More formal, neuropsychological testing should only be sought if there are clear abnormalities in terms of a patient's orientation (i.e. knowing the place, time, day, month), recall of recent events, or ability to do simple tests such as the reverse months (i.e. repeating all the months of the year in reverse order starting with December).

3.28 Are there tests you can do in the clinic that can confirm a diagnosis of anxiety?

There are no blood tests available for quick use in the clinic, but getting people to hyperventilate can be extremely informative. The simplest way to do this is to ask them to breathe at the same rate as oneself, and then start breathing quite quickly – say one to two breaths per second – and see how they react. Patients with anxiety disorders, especially those with a tendency to hyperventilate, will become quite anxious and even panicky within 20–30 seconds. Helping them to calm down, by getting them to take in long deep breaths, to hold each breath as long as possible, and then to breathe out very slowly, can also be instructive. In terms of panic syndrome and/or agoraphobia, a simple list of places or situations that they avoid (e.g. supermarkets, crowded shops, underground, bus, lift, train) when answered positively for more than two or three, is usually diagnostic.

While there are no definitive biochemical, haematological or radiological investigations diagnostic for anxiety or panic disorders, tests can of course exclude other illnesses and tend to get repeated because of patient demand. Research procedures indicate clear abnormalities of response in anxiety-prone patients, but these are not practical for clinical use. Thus, infusions of sodium lactate, or an alpha-2 agonist like yohimbine, or inspiration of CO_2, readily generates symptoms in 80–90% of patients, but in only 5% or less of controls. In other words, these disorders are certainly not all in the mind, and the possibilities for better management will be revolutionized when a reliable test comes along, as it surely will do.

3.29 Is anxiety associated with premenstrual tension (PMT)?

The typical symptom of PMT, in terms of the psychological symptoms, is irritability. This derives from a combination of physical discomfort, for example due to bloated breasts or abdomen, and a marked sense of inner tension. Patients also sleep badly, experience headaches, and can be readily sensitive to noise. This can lead to enhanced anxiety in terms of coping with social situations, dealing with difficult children, or relating to one's partner. There will also be a distinct pattern of such states of mind, the irritability/anxiety being very obvious for a few days prior to the period, and recurring on a monthly basis. Asking the patient to keep a simple mood diary ranging from +2 (feeling good, relaxed, cheerful) to −2 (feeling tense, edgy, irritable) can be quite helpful in clarifying matters.

3.30 What about other endocrine disorders like diabetes, Cushing's syndrome and/or Addison's disease, or phaeochromocytoma?

The only endocrine disorder that commonly presents with associated anxiety symptoms is thyrotoxicosis. There is no specific psychological syndrome associated with diabetes, apart from the confusion or even aggressive states of hypoglycaemia, while Cushing's syndrome and Addison's disease are strongly associated with depression rather than anxiety. That is to say, patients feel tired, slowed down, and lacking in drive, alongside their physical abnormalities. The extremely rare phaeochromocytoma (an adrenaline-secreting tumour of the adrenal gland) is regularly mentioned as a differential diagnosis of anxiety disorders and/or panic attacks, to the economic detriment of the many pathology laboratories asked to do VMA (vanillylmandelic acid) urine estimations. The key feature of this condition is that people develop sudden episodes of high blood pressure – something that does not occur in normal anxiety/panic attacks – and only that should be the trigger to further assessment. Endocrine disorders essentially have distinctive physical signs (e.g. striae in Cushing's syndrome), while the essence of anxiety states is their signlessness.

3.31 Are there any commonly prescribed medications that can lead to anxiety symptoms?

Yes. These are too numerous to mention all by name, and one should always closely question patients as to what drugs they are taking, illicit, recreational or prescribed. In terms of the latter, withdrawal from benzodiazepines, some antidepressants (there are several SSRIs such as paroxetine that have a distinct withdrawal syndrome), and other hypnotics can lead to anxiety states as well as impaired sleep. A range of other medications, for example steroids, beta stimulants, and SSRIs themselves can also cause distinct states of anxiety, particularly in those who are more anxiety prone anyway (*see Box 3.3*).

3.32 Can one readily differentiate between anxiety disorders and drug/alcohol withdrawal states?

This is a classic differential diagnostic problem, and often they are indistinguishable in presentation. Panic attacks are often part of alcohol

---

BOX 3.3 Drugs commonly associated with anxiety symptoms

Use of
- Caffeine
- β-stimulants, e.g. salbutamol
- Steroids
- Some SSRIs
- Cardiac medication, e.g. calcium-channel blockers and nitrates

Withdrawal from
- Alcohol
- Opiates
- Benzodiazepines
- Nicotine
- Barbiturates
- Some antidepressants, e.g. paroxetine
- Some antipsychotics

---

withdrawal, and patients with anxiety states, whether generalized anxiety, social phobia or agoraphobia, commonly turn to alcohol to alleviate their symptoms. Generally speaking an alcohol withdrawal state would be characterized by gross physical symptoms such as sweating and tremor, and if severe – moving on towards delirium tremens – visual hallucinations, for example of small animals, and even fits. Clearly a history of recent alcohol withdrawal, or recent drug use and withdrawal, will be vital in clarifying the cause of the anxiety/panic state. Furthermore, alcohol-induced panic will persist over a number of hours, and this is not the case for 'normal' panic attacks. Nevertheless, if in doubt it is best to assume the more serious diagnosis – of all the withdrawal states, alcohol withdrawal is the most dangerous – and treat as necessary (e.g. fluids, thiamine and benzodiazepines).

3.33 Where I can obtain help in getting diagnostic or assessment materials?

The Royal College of Psychiatrists (website: http://www.rcpsych.ac.uk/info/index.htm) publishes a number of pamphlets, which very nicely summarize the symptoms and treatment approaches for a range of conditions, including panic attacks, phobias, depression and anxiety in general. These also contain lists of useful books.

The *WHO Guide to Mental Health in Primary Care* (website: http://cebmh.warne.ox.ac.uk/cebmh/whoguidemhpcuk/) provides a mental disorder assessment guide, and there are also two standard assessment scales in Appendix 1 (*pp. 145–146*), namely the Hospital Anxiety and Depression Scale and the Impact of Event Scale.

PATIENT QUESTIONS

3.34   How can you be sure it is only anxiety?

The way anxiety presents, it is usually quite easy for a doctor to recognize it. There are experiences people have, phrases they use and the way they present their symptoms that fit with standard descriptions, and leaflets are available summarizing these. Sufferers certainly fear they may have a dangerous illness, but panic symptoms fade after a few minutes of self-relaxation, which does not happen in, for example, a heart attack or asthma attack. Use a questionnaire honestly on yourself and it is not difficult to recognize the problem.

3.35   Can anxiety cause cancer or other serious illnesses?

There is no evidence that anxiety causes cancer, although worrying about severe illnesses when you have unpleasant symptoms is quite understandable. There is also no association between getting cancer and feeling stressed or excessively anxious, although many people tend to look for possible reasons behind their own cancer. There is of course one exception to this rule, namely that smoking cigarettes regularly is the known cause of lung cancer, as well as of a number of other cancers. If you smoke to deal with anxiety, therefore, you are putting yourself at risk, as are all other smokers. Dealing with anxiety in a healthy way, via appropriate management, treatment or whatever – as outlined in this book – makes even more sense when you consider that sort of risk.

The aetiology of anxiety

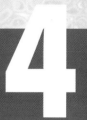

4.1 What is the mechanism behind feeling frightened when there is actually nothing to be frightened of?

This probably stems from an over-efficient evolutionary mechanism to ensure survival. The lifetime prevalence of anxiety disorders in general (20% or more) seems to show that we are better off being oversensitive than under-sensitive. The core feature of course is the 'fight or flight' response, which once triggered seems liable to be more easily triggered again in a given situation. Typically this would be in a crowded space, where patients describe an intrusive sense of being looked at, or when shortness of breath comes on after minor exertion. The process of 'kindling' in epilepsy, one fit lowering the threshold for another, may be a suitable analogy. The hypervigilance of anxiety reflects a failure to damp down the neurochemical arousal system, creating an especial sensitivity to anxiety cues or potential 'threats'.

4.2 Is there a known cause for anxiety disorders?

No single factor has been established as the cause of generalized anxiety, panic syndrome, or any of the related neuroses, such as depression or obsessive–compulsive disorder (OCD). However, anxiety does tend to run in families; genetic studies show that up to a third of first-degree relatives (i.e. mother or father, brother or sister, son or daughter) have a similar condition. This may of course present as mother having 'nerves', or as a brother being a heavy drinker or even drug abuser. There is also evidence that childhood anxiety, because of parental separation (about half of patients) or overprotective parenting, often seems to precede the adult condition. Some studies have shown that there are dependent personality traits in those who go on to develop anxiety disorders, but there is no set personality style that predicts who will become anxious in adulthood. Possible causes of anxiety disorder are summarized in *Box 4.1*.

4.3 Is it usually possible to highlight a particular patient's reason for developing a panic attack?

The first panic attack that a patient has, or at least in terms of what the patient describes in giving a history, will have occurred in a particular circumstance. Usually this will be in a crowded place, or in a tense social situation, or in the context of a depressive mood swing. Thus, it is perfectly possible to clarify exactly what happened when a particular patient had a panic attack, by the combination of observation and precise questioning (when did it happen? in what situation? was it crowded, e.g. store, bus, tube? any particular changes of habit in terms of diet, alcohol or other drinks recently?).

BOX 4.1 Possible causes of anxiety disorder

Biological
- In utero stress, e.g. maternal smoking
- Perinatal trauma/infection
- Head injury
- Hormonal conditions, e.g. thyrotoxicosis, phaeochromocytoma (very rare), carcinoid syndrome (very rare)
- Genetic inheritance

Psychosocial
- Childhood experience, e.g. abuse/bereavement
- Traumatic events
- Environmental, e.g. war/migration
- Family/cultural dysfunction

As often as not, however, panic attacks occur out of the blue. While there may be specific, understood reasons as to why a panic occurred, the ability to recognize such attacks as 'panic attacks' in itself is useful. But since we do not know what actually causes a panic attack (despite years of research) there is often a difficulty in clarifying causation for individual patients. The best approach is to ask a patient to keep a brief 'panic diary', noting when and where symptoms occur, what preceded them, and how long the panic lasted. This can also be the beginning of effective treatment, by enhancing insight, creating a therapeutic dialogue and setting up a system for monitoring symptoms and the course of the disorder.

INHERITED AND FAMILY FACTORS

4.4 Is there an inherited or genetic basis to anxiety and/or panic disorders?

The genetics of anxiety are well established. Not only does it tend to run in families, but there is a significant increase in concordance amongst monozygotic (i.e. identical) twins as compared to dizygotic (i.e. non-identical) twins. Thus something has been inherited to create such a difference, and this is borne out by the increased likelihood of first-degree and second-degree relatives having some form of anxiety. The problem is that such studies do not differentiate between different forms of anxiety, there being a 'spectrum' of neurotic disorders (anxiety, panic, depression, OCD), the particular type perhaps relating to a specific cause or age of onset. Some patients find it helpful to know that it is not really their fault that they are so troubled, while others find it hard to accept a physical basis for the way they feel. Understanding genetics should not preclude having an eclectic attitude to treatment, embracing psychological, pharmacological, and social approaches.

4.5   Does anxiety, or conditions like it, tend to run in families?

Yes, and strongly so. This may be inherited (*see Q. 4.4*), a learned behaviour, or a combination thereof. Different terms are often used for anxiety in different generations, such that an anxious individual may well describe her mother as having 'nerves' and her father as 'liking a drink'. It is unusual, by contrast, to have no evidence at all of anxiety being a family trait, and many families recognize their idiosyncrasies via nicknames or in-jokes. Such recognition can help in both diagnosis and reassurance.

4.6   Are there any particular problems in birth or childhood relevant to anxiety states?

There is some evidence that the combination of physical and sexual abuse in childhood is more likely to leave one suffering from a number of neurotic symptoms. This may well be physiologically induced, with identifiable brain changes on specific brain scans. It may in part be an inherited factor, since anxiety symptoms and alcohol abuse are commonly combined in those with the kind of limited impulse personalities that make up child abusers. More commonly, however, it is likely that an overanxious mother or father can lead to modelling by the child. Such overprotectiveness may lead to a kind of cotton wool effect whereby a child does not develop a natural range of activities and skills in dealing with the outside world. It does seem quite clear that anxious children are much more likely to become anxious adults, which is not surprising. Anxiety management should probably begin in schools.

4.7   What about the effects of abuse in childhood?

There is increasing evidence that physical and/or sexual abuse in childhood has physiological effects that can be picked up by sophisticated forms of brain scanning. Agoraphobia, with its underlying basis in anxiety, seems especially common in those who are known to have had such abuse at a young age. The obverse, that you are anxious probably because of such abuse does not, however, apply. There is also a theory (as yet unproven) suggesting that forms of viral infection in childhood can lead to significant changes, such as enhanced panic reactions. Of course, children learn to mimic their parents' reactions to events or symptoms, and this 'learned behaviour', in those who somatize, is likely to colour how patients present.

PSYCHOLOGICAL AND SOCIAL FACTORS

4.8 Are there any particular psychological theories that are relevant?

The models most commonly discussed are forms of learning theory and cognitive structuring. In the former, it is theorized that children/adolescents do learn from their parents, for example via conditioning (even though denying so) and model themselves in this way. They learn styles of coping, they pick up on the emotional tone of their families, and they learn to attribute symptoms or signs. Thus the notions of 'learned helplessness' and 'illness behaviour' (*Table 4.1*), the latter varying greatly from culture to culture.

> In terms of cognitive theory, it is considered that some individuals readily catastrophize what is going on. Thus they see a potentially anxiety-inducing situation, feel themselves becoming tense, tend to focus on worst-outcome scenarios, and reinforce their states of inner tension. Breaking up this pattern of thinking (cognitive behavioural therapy – *see Q. 7.6*) is therefore a way of improving self-control in anxiety. A tendency to over-inclusive thinking, being unable to exclude troubling thoughts or symptoms, is also common. The obsessional quality of many anxious patients is reflected in their repetitive questioning and inability to accept explanations.

4.9 Can particular events, like divorce or bereavement, or bad experiences, cause a formal anxiety disorder?

This is one of the big questions of research into anxiety, but unmasking of symptoms (i.e. no partner around to help) may be the key factor. There is

TABLE 4.1 Factors in illness behaviour (the way in which symptoms are understood and dealt with)

Factor	Example
Upbringing	Parental health style
Religion	Beliefs about causation
Social class	Knowledge and training
Gender	Attitudes to illness/pain
Age	Experience/lack of experience of symptoms
Culture	Accepted views of treatment needs
Work	Financial effects of illness

evidence that the first panic attack takes place in particularly distressing surroundings, for example a very crowded underground train or a packed supermarket. Whether this is merely the straw that breaks the camel's back, or causative in itself, is not known. Certain forms of anxiety disorder, for example post-traumatic stress disorder (PTSD), clearly arise from a more traumatic event, such as a frightening car crash. Such conditions will usually resolve within 3–6 months, and those who have persisting symptoms have almost always had a preceding tendency to anxiety/depression.

It is probably safer to say that there are degrees of vulnerability, and given enough shocks to the system, some people will develop formal anxiety states. It is perhaps more extraordinary to consider how many people do not develop such states, despite very frightening experiences. While many patients may prefer, and understand better, a social explanation, the fact is that the aetiology of anxiety disorders remains unclear.

4.10 Are there any known social or class factors more common in people with anxiety?

Overall it is accepted that anxiety/depressive disorders are more common in those of the so-called 'lower' social classes. This is reflected in terms of levels of smoking and alcohol use, in terms of presentations in primary care, and in terms of standard surveys, for example the General Health Questionnaire (GHQ). Furthermore, immigrant groups, depending on the reason for their emigration/immigration, can have higher rates of anxiety, possibly related to PTSD (because of traumatic experiences) or because of difficulties in cultural integration. The young, isolated, parentally non-supported, poor, and less well-educated individual is much more likely to develop a whole range of anxiety disorders. Given that about half of those with panic disorders have experienced some kind of parental separation in childhood, this may also reflect a degree of impaired personal education.

4.11 Is anxiety commoner in any particular social group?

There is no evidence that anxiety, as a disorder, is more prevalent amongst any particular society. It may show itself in more colourful ways in less sophisticated people, and it is accepted that younger women are more likely to bring their anxiety disorders to the attention of their doctor. Certain groups can be prone to 'group dynamics', particularly those in institutions, such as boarding schools or prisons. Attacks of fainting, or hoarseness, can spread very quickly, enhanced by the fear of a more serious underlying illness. Such episodes of 'mass hysteria' (now officially termed 'mass sociogenic illness') still occur, but seem to be less common now, perhaps owing to a more individualized style of living, or greater sophistication in health matters.

4.12 Is anxiety commoner in any particular cultural group?

The tendency to somatize conditions – to complain of physical problems rather than psychological concerns – has been associated with certain ethnic groups (e.g. South Asians, Chinese). But there is no evidence that these cultures have higher rates of anxiety or depression, while certain languages also lack many psychological terms. There are increased rates of a range of disorders in all those who have emigrated, particularly under unpleasant or threatening conditions, and disorders like PTSD, or even 'torture syndrome', include a number of anxiety symptoms. There are also different styles of presenting to the doctor, which may mimic a range of physical symptoms, and need to be understood as culturally generated. This is enhanced by the stigma of mental illness forcing people to avoid being categorized as 'mad' or 'weak-minded'.

4.13 Does anxiety present differently in people from different cultures?

There certainly are a wide range of presentations, in those of different genders, ages and cultures. A number of specific 'culture-bound' syndromes are very common. For example, so-called 'dhat' syndrome is the fear of loss of semen, well-recognized in certain groups of Indian males. The fear actually underlies a sense of tiredness and loss of energy that may go with a depressive illness, an anxiety disorder, or even panic attacks. The GP needs to go beneath the presentation to ask specific questions about specific symptoms. Conditions like 'koro' (fear of losing one's penis) in South East Asian, usually Chinese, older males, or of 'latah' in South East Asian women (automatic obedience, etc.) are similar types of presentation. In fact most cultures have a word, or group of words, to describe the sense of loss, lack of control, tiredness or despair that may be the presenting feature of an anxiety/depressive condition (*Table 4.2*).

4.14 Is there any specific association between immigration and anxiety?

This would depend on the reasons for the immigration, and the circumstances in which the immigrants find themselves. By and large all immigrant groups have increased rates of psychiatric disorder, whether it be formal schizophrenic illnesses or the milder forms of anxiety. Isolation can lead to considerable depressive feelings, readily compounded by racist attitudes, poor language skills, or a history of abuse or assault in the country from which the person has come.

TABLE 4.2 Culture-bound symptoms associated with anxiety states

Name	Region/country	Symptoms
Koro	East Asia	Fear of the penis disappearing into one's body, resulting in death
Latah Imu	South East Asia Japan	States of automatic obedience, copying acts and words, however inappropriate (or even obscene)
Dhat Shenkui	India China	Symptoms such as anxiety, fatigue, weakness, dizziness, attributed to a feared excessive loss of semen
Hwa-Byung	Korea	Anxiety symptoms such as panic, insomnia, indigestion and palpitations attributed to suppressed anger
Nerva	Greece	Multi-symptom presentation including insomnia, anxiety, headaches, poor concentration and indigestion related to life stresses
Brain fag	West Africa	Impaired concentration, tiredness, headache, visual disturbances and a sense of physical pressure on the head

Some immigrants may of course be feeling so relieved at coming to a safe place, away from the threats and deprivations of the home country, that they may be remarkably phlegmatic despite all of their problems, limited social and financial circumstances, and unpleasant memories. As often as not it is the personal circumstances in which they find themselves, for example cramped and crowded rooms, in temporary hostels, that are as much part of the problem as any formal illness.

PHYSICAL FACTORS

4.15 Is anxiety a biochemical condition?

The answer is almost certainly yes, in the light of current research. Given the nature of the symptoms that patients experience, and their similarities to the 'fight or flight' response, an overactive adrenaline/noradrenaline system seems the obvious mechanism. Unfortunately, there is no evidence of increased levels of any neurochemical in anxiety/panic patients, although they are

> overreactive when given specific stimulants such as sodium lactate. Thus, measures of forearm blood flow or eye mydriasis show enhancement and prolongation of effect, even after the stimulus (i.e. a lactate infusion) has been discontinued.

It is also clear that effective medication seems to work by *increasing* monoamine activity, whether noradrenaline, adrenaline or serotonin, which is something of a paradox. This could be explained by neurochemicals having different effects at different brain regions, or by anomalies of receptor reactivity. Increasingly, research has focused on the role of gamma-aminobutyric acid (GABA), a substance that seems to damp down neuronal activity as a balance to the arousing effects of serotonin or noradrenaline. Such an underactive GABA-ergic system would explain the nicely calming effects of both benzodiazepines and alcohol, since they directly stimulate GABA receptors. By contrast, a number of regularly prescribed medications can cause anxiety symptoms, probably acting via similar mechanisms (*see Table 4.3*).

4.16 Is anxiety a hormonal condition?

Probably not. There is as yet no evidence of any detectable hormonal abnormality, although there is a detailed literature on cortisol hyperreactivity in major depressive illness. Growth hormone (GH) and prolactin responses to specific serotoninergic or noradrenergic probes have been used to monitor activity, but apart from hyperthyroidism there is no association between endocrine disorders (e.g. acromegaly, Cushing's syndrome) and anxiety/panic syndromes.

In the differential diagnosis of anxiety, the elimination of thyroid overactivity, which often presents with palpitations or sweating, may of

TABLE 4.3 Drugs that may cause anxiety or anxiety-like symptoms	
Stimulants	Caffeine, aminophylline, theophylline, cocaine, amfetamines
Anticholinergics	Procyclidine, benzhexol, oxybutynin
Sympathomimetics	Ephedrin, pseudoephedrine, phenylpropanolamine
Dopaminergics	Bromocriptine, L-dopa
Withdrawal	Alcohol, benzodiazepines, opiates
Others	Steroids, hallucinogens, e.g. LSD, ecstasy, baclofen

course be a most important investigation. Rare conditions such as phaeochromocytoma should not be considered unless there are striking physical signs (e.g. acutely raised blood pressure – *see Q. 3.30*).

4.17 Is anxiety commoner in those who have been assaulted or had a traffic accident?

There is an association between depressive illnesses and life events, but the combination of shock and physical injury that goes with assaults or traffic accidents can produce a range of problems. Any form of concussion, even the briefest loss of consciousness, can be associated with so-called 'post-concussional' states. These are unpleasant conditions characterized by loss of concentration, a sense of tiredness, dizzy spells and headaches, social withdrawal, enhanced irritability, and other mood changes. They can go on for 2 or 3 years, particularly if there has been a significant concussive event.

Likewise, after traffic accidents, up to 15% of people will experience a form of post-traumatic stress disorder (PTSD), or travel anxiety/phobia. This is usually because of the circumstances of the accident, in that victims have *not* lost consciousness at all and have therefore been witness to everything. Being trapped in a car, seeing unpleasant sights (i.e. dead bodies, blood, piles of wreckage) or having genuinely been put at risk of death, are common factors. Such conditions last between 3 and 6 months, usually, and are characterized by persistent flashbacks, nightmares and disturbed sleep, being very jumpy and arousable, mood changes, and/or feeling somewhat 'numbed' by the whole experience. Such reactions come with varying degrees of intensity, sometimes as a brief stress reaction, for a few days, sometimes in a more prolonged way, evolving even into a chronic depression.

Assaults or traffic accidents, or similar frightening incidents, can also lead to avoidance and a formal 'travel phobia'. People will develop an irrational fear of the situation that led to the fear (i.e. travelling in a car), be aware that the fear is irrational, but be unable to control it. Some will never travel in a car again, or at least never drive one. They will have enhanced anxiety symptoms, being 'impossible' back-seat drivers, being very jittery, and sometimes getting panic attacks and even jumping out of cars at the slightest opportunity. These conditions are poorly understood and often missed, not least because people are too embarrassed to tell GPs about them. Contacting a family member can be most illuminating.

4.18 Can head injuries cause enhanced anxiety?

Unfortunately, head injury can lead to virtually any symptom or abnormal behaviour, depending on the circumstance, the site of the injury, the extent of the damage and one's premorbid personality. Damage to specific areas of the brain (e.g. frontal lobe) has well-defined consequences, but nonlocalized head injuries, particularly when the person has been in a coma, can often lead to an apparent 'change of personality'.

Specifically, the individual becomes rather more irritable, sometimes more paranoid, more socially withdrawn and even a caricature of his or her former self. Anxiety symptoms will emerge in the context of a number of such presentations, either because of the fear that one will not recover, or as part and parcel of a direct response. Again, excessive use of alcohol is not uncommon, and this can compound a range of symptoms, particularly irritability, social anxiety, and post-concussional states (*see* Q. 4.17).

DRUG EFFECTS

4.19 Does alcohol make anxiety better or worse?

Alcohol is one of the best anxiolytics there is, and has been used for centuries in this role. It is remarkably effective in helping shy people socialize, in relaxing after a specific stress, or in getting one off to sleep. Used sensibly, as most people try to do, it is a safe form of self-medication. The problem for those suffering from morbid anxiety, or panic attacks, is that it very quickly can become a regular habit. Such individuals will also suffer tolerance, that is the need to drink more alcohol to ensure they get anxiety relief.

It is probably true to say that most people suffering from alcohol dependence, do, in fact, have some underlying form of enhanced arousal, whether presenting as anxiety, panic attacks, social clumsiness or lowered self-esteem. It is often difficult to tell, with older patients (i.e. in their 40s and 50s), which came first, the anxiety or the alcohol problem. Anyone presenting with obvious signs of anxiety should of course be closely checked for symptoms of alcohol dependence or withdrawal.

4.20 Does smoking cigarettes have an effect on anxiety states?

The extraordinary power of nicotine is its ability to stimulate concentration in those feeling tired or slowed down, but to relax those feeling stressed or tense. It is this double ability that makes it so addictive, and one does not need to be a historian to understand why smoking was taken up so widely during the Second World War. Smoking therefore does relieve anxiety, for many people, and the widespread nature of the habit indicates how widespread are anxiety states of a milder form. It is also probably true that smoking, like drinking alcohol, lowers the threshold to developing minor anxiety symptoms, in a somewhat vicious circle of tension and dependence. Coming off nicotine, therefore, always enhances anxiety, symptoms like muscle tension, irritability and difficulty in concentrating being especially prominent.

4.21 Are illicit drugs an important factor in generating anxiety problems?

Illicit drugs in themselves are usually taken as anxiety relief. That is particularly so in the case of opiates (i.e. heroin, morphine) or cannabis, and withdrawal from these often creates anxiety/panic symptoms. More stimulant drugs like amfetamines or cocaine can have a 'paradoxical' effect in some people, in that they may actually make them feel calm, but by and large they are used to stimulate and enhance sensations. In this sense they can create quite intense levels of anxiety, either via forms of paranoia (e.g. with amfetamines) or because of unpleasant side-effects like palpitations or headaches. The hallucinogenic properties of drugs such as LSD can make people intensely panicky, and the use of benzodiazepines in such individuals is often remarkably, and quickly, effective. The phrase 'freaking out' neatly represents what could more formally be called 'drug-induced anxiety'.

LIFESTYLE OR OCCUPATIONAL STRESS

4.22 What is the best way of defining stress?

The term 'stress' is widely used, and is popularly thought to have a specific diagnostic status, which it does not have. It probably has at least two core meanings, namely that uncomfortable state of mind due to the perception of not being able to cope, and the consequences of that state of mind (i.e. headaches, shakiness, lowered mood). If patients complain of stress one should ask them just what they mean by that, and get them to describe just what specific symptoms they are having, or what specific problems they are finding it difficult to cope with. Terms such as 'work stress' are very poorly defined, whereas PTSD (post-traumatic stress disorder) is quite closely defined (*see Q. 5.18*). It is also worth remembering that one person's stress factor might be another's thrill factor, for example driving fast or handling crises at work, although the physiology of the stress response (release of adrenaline and corticosteroids) is well established (*Fig. 4.1*).

4.23 Are anxiety problems caused by 'stress'?

This is probably true, but not necessarily true. It is likely that the 'stress' that the patient is complaining of is, in fact, the anxiety disorder itself, for example panic attacks. Whenever patients complain of stress, it is worth exploring just what that word means to them, and worth clarifying the actual symptoms that are being experienced. Clearly someone who has been

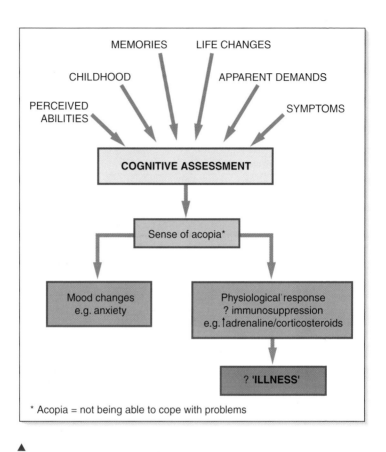

Fig. 4.1 A cognitive stress model.

through a difficult time, for example at work or at home, is more likely to complain of problems, and if that person suffers from anxiety symptoms, or even physical symptoms with an anxiety component (e.g. palpitations) these are all likely to be exacerbated. The fact of the matter is that it takes a combination of untoward events and impaired personal resilience to unmask anxiety, and if the patient wants an explanation in terms of the stress/social impact model, then that can be helpful in promoting treatment compliance.

4.24 Are there any particular jobs associated with higher levels of anxiety?

It is often assumed that there are greater levels of 'stress' in particular jobs, for example teaching, working in high-powered and fast-moving environments (i.e. the stock exchange) or working in the police with its attendant risks. Certainly a number of individuals are now presenting with work-related 'stress', but this has a range of components. If patients are worrying about their job, or feeling 'stressed out' by it, with typical anxiety symptoms, it may well be that there is an underlying/depressive disorder which has been attributed to work. Clearly there are specific situations, i.e. threats of redundancy or bullying, which can lead people to attend the doctor more often, but studies usually show that it is the unemployed who see the doctor more often than the employed. Self-report surveys of workplace stress are difficult to evaluate, reflecting job satisfaction and pay as much as any significant illness. Sickness rates are in fact used by personnel departments as an index of management competence.

4.25 Should anxious patients be advised to take time off work?

GPs are often asked for their advice as to whether people should go back to work, take up a new job, etc., and it is tempting to try to help. But symptoms of an anxiety disorder do not necessarily mean that the person affected will not be able to function at work, and many in fact feel better off within the routines of work (provided they can get there). As always, it will depend on the nature of the symptoms, the individual's own reaction to them, and the working environment. The inability to cope with the job in hand, i.e. being promoted beyond one's abilities, is sadly a common problem ('the Peter principle'), and a long-standing source of vexation to the average personnel manager. There is considerable expertise within the occupational health speciality, whose advice should be sought in such a context.

4.26 Is anxiety due to modern lifestyles?

Urban environments create more possibilities for anxiety or phobic symptoms to emerge, by virtue of their crowds, noise, travel arrangements and cheek-by-jowl housing. It is difficult to have agoraphobia when living in rural isolation, although that may be the reason some folk choose to live there. Likewise pressured work, stimulant drugs (coffee as much as cocaine), lack of sleep and lifestyle assumptions create casualties of expectation. Getting patients to go through a typical day can be most helpful in clarifying perceived stress factors in anxiety.

4.27 Can environmental factors, such as pollution, climate or altitude, cause anxiety disorders?

No association has to date been established with any overt environmental factor. The wise physician will of course never exclude unusual possibilities; for example, toxins from industrial effluent creating a variety of symptom patterns, psychological and physical. To misquote Oscar Wilde, to miss one patient's mercury poisoning is unfortunate, to miss two (or a whole township's) sounds like carelessness.

In terms of climate, there is an increased incidence of seasonal affective disorder syndrome (SADS) in those living in higher latitudes, which is thought to be due to light deficiency. Essentially a depressive illness, it may sometimes present with anxiety symptoms. There are also the known pulmonary effects of high altitude, with confusional states not uncommon in mountain climbers. Mildly hypomanic states, with enhanced anxiety, have also been reported.

4.28 Are there any particular foods or dietary factors behind anxiety?

Despite extensive research there is no evidence that any specific food, or diet (e.g. vegetarian, organic) can worsen or improve an anxiety disorder. Many alternative practitioners suggest certain approaches, for example a milk-free diet for those with chronic catarrh, or diets designed to avoid certain foodstuffs. The excessive use of caffeine, in coffee, tea or even chocolate, as well as in diet colas, can lead to some people developing obvious symptoms of over-arousal. These would include feeling sweaty and having palpitations, and not sleeping. It is always worth checking with patients just what they are eating, and whether they do have any specific fads, because there can be some strange patterns unearthed, and people may reject taking their medication. Many patients also prefer to take health products, of whatever sort, rather than 'pills', but by and large such products are harmless, and rarely enhance (or genuinely alleviate) anxiety. Vitamin deficiency conditions that are rare today (e.g. pellagra, due to niacin deficiency) can present with psychological effects.

4.29 Does lack of serotonin cause anxiety?

While specific serotonin reuptake inhibitors (SSRIs) seem to be effective in treating some patients, there is no reliable evidence that anxious patients have low serotonin levels. Post-mortem studies of those committing suicide have shown possible reduced serotonin activity in the frontal lobes, but this seems related to depressive and impulse-control symptoms, not enhanced anxiety. There is also no evidence that increased serotonin intake (e.g. in bananas) alleviates anxiety, although SSRIs often cause/enhance anxiety symptoms when taken initially. Some patients are unable to tolerate them at all because of this somewhat paradoxical effect.

4.30 Does shyness or lowered self-esteem cause anxiety disorders?

These states of mind may often seem to be part of an anxiety disorder, enhancing the effect of symptoms, but do not seem to be a direct cause. They are also more often associated with *social phobia*. This is characterized by a persisting fear of social interaction, whether something as simple as going out on a date, or more demanding, such as speaking in public. Blushing, sweating and a dry mouth are typical symptoms, and many 'shy' people are to all intents and purposes socially phobic. While symptoms do overlap it is worth pursuing the background details of such individuals since a different treatment approach may be needed.

4.31 Are there any good analogies for anxiety/panic attacks to help clarify matters to patients?

A useful analogy is the notion of an oversensitive car alarm. Thus an anxious patient can be seen as suffering from the kind of alarm system that fires off when only a leaf, say, has floated down and set off the mechanism. A particularly annoying and oversensitive smoke alarm (e.g. at work) or fire alarm (on a neighbour's house) can also be used to draw the analogy. In this way patients can be complimented on their being 'more sensitive' than others, as well as helped to consider that they are not 'mad' or going mad. The 'wiring' metaphor can be extended to further consultations, to help people understand the nature of their condition (it is a 'real' illness, not just in your mind) and ways to 'repair' it.

Another approach for those with prominent chest/dyspnoeic symptoms is to use the analogy of being suffocated. It is as if all the air has been sucked out of the room, and patients feel they are being smothered in their sleep (panic attacks often occurring in the night). The state of fear induced by scary horror movies, in which heroines pant, cry, shake and faint, may also be useful given the visual images evoked.

4.32 Why does anxiety come back again after it seems to have resolved?

Generalized anxiety disorder tends to be a chronic condition, with relapses and remissions over the years. An illness, a stressful event or bereavement, or even some random memory (i.e. seeing a divorced partner in a shopping centre) may trigger things off. Anxiety-prone people tend to find it difficult to put troubling thoughts or concerns out of their minds, thus the effectiveness of cognitive behavioural therapy (CBT – *see Q. 7.6*), both in dealing with the condition and in prolonging the effects of drug treatment.

As often as not, discontinuation of effective medication will be a factor. The patient may have successfully come off a benzodiazepine or antidepressants some months earlier, and have stayed apparently well for that time. Regular relapses may mean maintenance medication will be required.

 PATIENT QUESTIONS

4.33 Is anxiety caused by the way you are brought up?

It is difficult to establish whether a particular type of childhood or parenting approach causes people to be anxious. It is known that children who lose a parent when young (i.e. when they are under 10 years old) are more likely to be depressed in later life, and depression often has anxiety as part of the symptoms. It is also known that worried parents tend to have worried children, habits passed on as a mixture of copying your mother's (or father's) way of doing things. You also inherit, perhaps, their kind of metabolism. Smoking and drinking patterns tend to run in families, and are usually ways of dealing with feeling tense or nervous. Of course having an anxious parent can be useful, in that you may be able to learn from them how to cope with anxiety symptoms.

4.34 Is anxiety genetic?

Anxiety, or 'nerves', or something like the two, does seem to run in families, but the basis is not clear. It may just be a tendency to worry too much, or it may be because we all tend to take on some of our parents' styles of doing things. Most people who have anxiety symptoms, of whatever form, can often remember someone in their family tree – an aunt or uncle, or a grandparent – who seemed to be a little bit troubled or nervous, or perhaps drank a bit too much. Increasing research has shown these kinds of inherited patterns, and if there is someone in your family who fits the bill, then this is a kind of reassurance that it is not unlikely that anxiety is your problem. But the chances still remain very high (80% or more) that most of your children will not suffer, so fears of passing on some bad inheritance are not worth holding to. This genetic connection, of course, is making us understand much more about how anxiety affects people, has helped with developing new treatments, and is likely to help with getting new treatments going in the future.

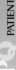 PATIENT QUESTIONS

EDUCATION CENTRE LIBRARY
FURNESS GENERAL HOSPITAL
BARROW-IN-FURNESS

Anxiety and ~~associated~~ psychiatric conditions

5

5.1 What is the difference between anxiety neurosis, neurasthenia, generalized anxiety disorder and panic disorder?

There is probably considerable overlap, but essentially these terms reflect historical patterns of understanding. 'Anxiety neurosis' was a term coined by Sigmund Freud, to describe patients with a mixture of anxiety and panic symptoms that he deemed to derive from aspects of childhood sexuality. Neurasthenia was a 19th century term, embracing depressive and anxiety symptoms, and thought to be due to a 'weakness' of the nervous system, requiring strengthening medications. It is now best considered as an old-fashioned term for chronic fatigue syndrome (ME).

The modern terms, 'generalized anxiety disorder' and 'panic disorder' embrace overlapping entities, the former comprising a persistent sense of worry, restlessness and irritability, difficulties concentrating and sleeping, associated depression, and a chronic tendency. The latter embraces the distinct phenomenon of formal, 'out of the blue' panic attacks (*see Ch. 3*) which does seem to be different in terms of some brain mechanisms, biological reactions and particular cognitive attitudes. Thus panic patients tend to 'catastrophize' readily, when confronted by physical symptoms for example, and seem to respond better to different treatment approaches. A wide range of terms, however, is still used, which is muddling for patients, families and practitioners.

5.2 What is meant by agoraphobia?

This is, literally, a fear of the marketplace (transcribing the Greek original) but it is *not* a fear of open places. Like all phobias it is a fear out of proportion to the actual threat, known to be so by the sufferer, yet creating avoidance of the feared situation. Sufferers either avoid going out altogether, or only go out accompanied, or have a very limited range of places (i.e. the corner shop for less than 5 minutes) that they will go to. Supermarkets, the underground, trains and buses (especially if crowded) are all anathema, being associated with panic symptoms and unpleasant experiences. As a result patients tend to use cars or taxis for minor journeys, visit parks to walk the dog in the quiet of the early evening, or only visit empty shops – 24-hour supermarkets are an agoraphobic goldmine – so as to alleviate their sense of being trapped. Agoraphobia is best understood as a behavioural response to panic attacks, rather than an 'illness' in itself, despite its textbook classification.

5.3 Do all people suffering with anxiety disorder also have agoraphobia?

No. Most patients with generalized anxiety disorder can go out independently, and many have no limitations in how often they go out or where they go. Many are, however, sensitive to certain situations, especially closed-in places such as lifts or the underground. In assessing patients it is important to inquire about agoraphobia, which is best seen as a behavioural response to anxiety and/or panic episodes. Because patients do not have agoraphobia does not mean they do not suffer significantly from chronic anxiety symptoms. These may primarily affect their interpersonal behaviour, social relationships, and family or work situations, or even emerge in terms of chronic physical symptoms like irritable bowel syndrome.

5.4 Is agoraphobia always due to anxiety or panic attacks?

Anxiety and panic disorder, the latter especially, are the common causes of agoraphobia, but other underlying conditions may create a behavioural pattern that seems very similar to agoraphobia. Thus, withdrawn sensitive individuals, with so-called avoidant or schizotypal personality disorders, will simply avoid crowded places because they do not like being with people. Cultural factors, such as religious limitations or the fears associated with uncertain immigrant status, can also lead to social avoidance, as can the consequences of a serious or dangerous accident or shock (e.g. post-traumatic stress disorder). Other causes of an apparent agoraphobia include depression, in which the patient simply cannot be bothered, or lacks the energy, to go out, or paranoid psychotic states, in which people believe they are being harassed, followed, spied upon or interfered with, and thus they stay indoors, even covering up the windows with blankets. It is also worth considering that some people actually do not like shopping.

5.5 Is anxiety often associated with social phobia?

Social phobia can be considered as a distinct form of anxiety disorder, generated by a fear of public scrutiny and possible humiliation in public places. Sufferers tend in particular to have physical symptoms such as blushing, dry mouth, sweaty palms, and tremor. Public speaking, initiating conversations, especially with strangers, or going out on a date, are particular problems. Such patients can be distinguished from those with panic disorder by their preferring to go out alone, rather than accompanied, and by preferring, for example, to sit with their back to the wall in a room rather than near the door. The panic patient needs the door because a quick exit may be needed. By contrast with generalized anxiety, however, socially phobic patients should not experience significant anxiety symptoms outside of their socially troubling situations, although many do have co-morbid anxiety and/or depressive illnesses as well.

5.6 Is there a particular pattern of mixed anxiety/depression that makes it a distinct condition?

This category remains a real problem in terms of both diagnosis and management, not least because patients tend to change over time. Thus there is the concept of 'the neurotic spectrum', someone seeming predominantly anxious at a consultation, and 3 months later, for example, seeming to be rather low, depressed and tearful. Social factors may be important in generating different responses, and in older people agitated depression is often misinterpreted as only being anxiety, with a failure to give an appropriate antidepressant. By and large, however, mixed anxiety and depression, whichever the predominant presentation, responds to the same medication, and can also be helped by specific psychological approaches.

5.7 Is there a real difference between anxiety and milder forms of depression?

A number of depressed patients do not feel anxious, their key symptoms being those of tiredness, impaired drive and concentration, and a rather hopeless/helpless outlook. In this sense they do differ from those with mild anxiety, although there is considerable overlap. Both groups of patients tend to somatize, especially if particularly concerned, personally or culturally, about the stigma attached to psychiatric terminology. Clarifying and monitoring an individual patient's specific symptoms is probably more useful, in many cases, than worrying as to whether anxiety or depression is the 'correct' diagnosis.

5.8 What does the word 'neurosis' actually mean?

By definition the 'neuroses' are forms of mental illness in which patients remain in touch with reality. That is to say they do not experience hallucinations (perceptions in the absence of a stimulus, for example hearing voices that no one else can hear), nor do they suffer from deluded thinking or formal thought disorder, both of which prevent one making sense of what is happening in the world around. Neuroses can therefore be contrasted, in psychiatry generally, with the 'psychoses', the latter including schizophrenia and manic depression.

The major neuroses are anxiety, depression, panic syndrome, social phobia, post-traumatic stress disorder and obsessive–compulsive disorder. They are currently assumed to derive as much from social factors and relationship problems, as from problems of brain wiring, although research increasingly shows that neurochemical abnormalities, and differential responses on specialized brain scans, also underlie many of these conditions.

The term 'neurotic', while technically value-neutral, has become associated with a denigratory attitude towards some patients, alongside phrases such as 'the walking worried'. Distinguishing neurotic illnesses (i.e. neuroses) from neurotic personalities can be very difficult of course. But if patients have a distinct pattern of symptoms, as outlined in the categories discussed in this chapter, then it is fair to consider that they do have a potentially treatable illness.

5.9 What are the key symptoms of obsessive–compulsive disorder (OCD)?

Obsessions are recurrent, unwanted thoughts, that patients know to be silly, but simply cannot put out of their head. Compulsions are the actions taken, often in the form of rituals (e.g. hand washing) to relieve the anxiety generated by these thoughts, for example fears of contamination. Because of this pattern of thinking and behaving, OCD sufferers may spend hours of their day in complex washing rituals, preparation rituals, or avoidance rituals. Milder forms of presentation include patients who regularly clean and dust their houses (i.e. are 'house-proud') or whose obsessional traits make them very careful and punctilious in their daily dealings. Paradoxically, the most severely affected will often live in considerable dirt and chaos, being so trapped by their symptoms that they cannot even face the complexity of actions involved, even in getting out of bed.

5.10 Are anxiety and OCD symptoms often found together?

While most patients with anxiety disorder do not have OCD, most OCD patients do have a tendency to worry, around specific issues associated with their obsession. The diagnosis may even be missed, because of what seem to be obvious anxiety or even depressive symptoms, if one does not ask specifically for obsessional patterns of thinking. People are embarrassed to discuss these, but are often very relieved to be able to tell someone when asked. Like anxiety, OCD can respond well to forms of cognitive and/or cognitive behavioural intervention, as well as SSRIs, particularly in higher doses.

5.11 What is meant by the term 'dysthymia'?

This term has largely replaced the outdated concept of 'neurotic depression', and is best understood as a form of chronic, mild, but nevertheless intrusive depression. Lifetime prevalence rates are around 5%, and it is twice as common in women. Depressive symptoms are constant, do not quite amount to what is termed 'moderate or major depression', but may lead on to more serious forms of depression in later life. Typical symptoms include difficulty remembering all the symptoms one has had over the last 2 years, indecisiveness, feelings of inferiority and guilt, impaired self-confidence, and even decreased libido.

As a result, work and social performance are impaired, patients feel very distressed at their own incapacities, and patients regularly seek prolonged courses of treatment. There tends to be a considerable overlap with anxiety and OCD, as well as with substance abuse, whether cannabis, tranquillizers or alcohol. It is probably best considered as a subcategory of a chronic type of the depressive spectrum. Patients often require high-dose treatments, for quite a long period of time.

5.12 Is anxiety described quite differently in other cultures?

By and large anxiety has similar symptoms the world over, but the English language is blessed – or cursed? – by having many psychological terms to describe subtleties of the experience. Many patients, particularly from the Third World, will simply describe heart symptoms or headaches, and there are a range of specific terms used depending on where one comes from. In Japanese for example the term 'shinkei-shitsu' describes an intense embarrassment on looking at other people, while 'putzwut' is a cleaning madness described in parts of Switzerland. No matter the term used, one can often establish the core symptoms, for example of palpitations or feeling panicky in public places, despite the tendency for many such patients to somatize. A number of the more common 'culture-bound syndromes' are to be found in *Table 4.2*.

5.13 What is meant by the koro syndrome?

This is a form of anxiety, often accompanied by a number of physical symptoms such as palpitations or nausea, that seems particularly associated with a fear of penile retraction in older males. It is strongly linked with fears of impotence and physical decline, and was originally described in Chinese males from South East Asia. It has increasingly been described in European cultures, and there are arguments as to whether it is a form of depression or something quite specific. It is probably best seen as a symptom of anxiety or panic disorder, and treated as such.

5.14 Does alcohol dependence often arise out of anxiety?

Alcohol is an excellent tranquillizer, and there is no doubt that many patients with alcohol-dependent characteristics will describe a sense of their social anxiety being relieved when they drink alcohol. In this sense many alcoholics were socially phobic, needing alcohol to give them social courage and to make themselves feel interesting to other people. There is no distinct pattern of personality style, however, related to alcohol dependence, and there is no evidence whatsoever of a formal dependent or addictive personality disorder. The similarities of course between alcohol withdrawal and forms of panic disorder are noteworthy, and there is some evidence that reduced craving can be secondary to giving SSRIs. Alcoholism in general, however, probably arises out of a complex pattern of social, family and personal characteristics.

5.15 What are the commonest drugs people take to deal with anxiety?

Alcohol is the universal tranquillizer, widely used and abused. The next most common anxiety reliever of choice is probably nicotine, with its strange ability to calm the anxious and yet enhance the concentration of those feeling tired and run-down. This is probably the basis for its powerful addictive properties. All drugs that reduce anxiety, for example benzodiazepines or barbiturates, by definition make people feel better, even slightly euphoric, and thus are addictive. Some patients, however, dislike the idea of being drugged or artificially calmed down, and may even feel more anxious at the impairments generated by such medication. Paradoxically a number of patients report feeling calmer on caffeine, or even cocaine. The increasing use of cannabis in modern society as a general tranquillizer, muscle relaxant and sleep enhancer reflects how many different forms of drug can be of help to people suffering from anxiety.

5.16 Do people with anxiety disorders more commonly use opiates, or cannabis?

There is no clear evidence that generalized anxiety disorder or panic syndrome, or even social phobia, are the basis for developing dependence on opiates or associated drugs. There is also no good evidence that opiates significantly reduce panic attacks, unless these are part of an opiate withdrawal syndrome. It may be, however, that those with an anxiety disorder who also become addicted to opiates would be more sensitive to withdrawal symptoms, and thus be more liable to remain addicted. A particular problem in researching the basis for addictions is that clarifying premorbid personality styles or illnesses, retrospectively, can be very difficult.

5.17 Is it common for anxious patients to resort to stimulant drugs like cocaine or amfetamines?

This is unusual, since symptoms are worsened, but there is no doubt that a number of patients report paradoxical effects from stimulants. Amfetamines thus make them feel subjectively calmer, even though they may be more active and sleep less. Similarly, although cannabis is generally seen as a tranquillizer, a number of individuals find it makes them aroused and even 'paranoid' and thus avoid it. The general rule is that people do not generally take things that make them feel worse, but there is no fixed pattern of premorbid personality, or level of anxiety, that predicts what drug anyone will become addicted to.

5.18 What is meant by post-traumatic stress disorder (PTSD)?

PTSD is a pattern of symptoms that result from an extremely traumatizing event, such as an assault or traffic accident. This event will normally have put one into fear for one's life. Patients tend to re-experience the event, seeing it in their mind's eye, have flashbacks or dreams about the event, often of a nightmarish quality, avoid anything that might remind them of the event (e.g. driving), and are over-aroused and hypervigilant, reacting to noise, and withdrawing socially. Symptoms usually last for at least 3 if not 6 months, or even more, but then gradually resolve with or without treatment. There is evidence that medication (e.g. SSRIs) can be helpful, but no evidence that counselling is effective. Research has shown that those who are more anxiety prone or of an obsessional disposition are likely to suffer such symptoms.

5.19 What is meant by an acute stress disorder?

This is the response to a severe life-threatening event, as in PTSD, that occurs briefly for days, or a week or two after an accident. Flashbacks, bad dreams, impaired sleep and tearfulness, as a reaction to the event, can generally be seen as understandable. Its quick resolution usually means that treatment is not required, apart from perhaps sleeping medication for a short while.

5.20 Is anxiety the common cause of 'hysterical' reactions?

This may seem so, but will depend on one's definition of 'hysteria'. This is now an outdated term, although popularly used. Technically it embraces the behaviour generated by the unconscious 'conversion' of psychological anxiety into a physical symptom, for example an inability to speak or an apparent hemiplegia. Such reactions are usually accompanied by an oddly un-anxious state, 'la belle indifférence'.

Anxiety may be much more relevant in cases of 'mass hysteria' (mass sociogenic illness). This is uncommon now, but represents the adoption of a particular symptom or set of symptoms by a group, often children in a school or other institutionalized people. A dominant core group will start the process, and historical examples abound, for example witchcraft trials.

5.21 What is meant by terms like 'dissociation' and 'conversion'?

These are both processes associated with hysterical reactions (*see* Q. 5.20). In the former, one adopts a separate personality, unconsciously, and individuals sometimes spend days in a dissociative fugue, doing normal day-to-day tasks (e.g. driving, going to shops) but subsequently having no recall of what they have done or where they have been. Conversion involves a more specific reaction, developing a physical symptom due to psychological anxiety. It is often confused with malingering, because of the concept of 'secondary gain' whereby individuals generate sympathy, support or a change in reaction to them because of their hysterical state. Recent research seems to show a genuine neurological basis, but this remains controversial.

5.22 Is impotence in middle-aged men really due to psychological reasons like anxiety?

Anxiety and depression, even the notion of a male menopause, have been seen as the typical bases of impotence, but modern research has shown, however, that increasing numbers of impotence cases are based on a physical problem, whether it be diabetes, hypertension, other forms of vascular disease or hormonal conditions. Alcohol or drug excess can also be significant. The development of 'wonder' drugs like sildenafil (Viagra) has in particular enhanced the biological/physical approach. Nevertheless, performance anxiety should not be dismissed, particularly in a climate where expectations of male sexual function continue to outweigh the realities of physiological ability. Despite macho claims, research studying the sexual behaviour of Mediterranean males has shown that the great majority rarely have an orgasm more than two or three times a week.

5.23 Can anxiety actually cause premature ejaculation (in men) or anorgasmia (in women)?

These two conditions are the commonest forms of sexual disorder, and are certainly worsened by states of anxiety or depression. By and large both respond, however, to sensitive forms of sexual therapy, such as the 'squeeze' technique for men, and the need for greater sexual education as to approaches to foreplay and differential expectations. Treatment of an underlying anxiety or panic disorder is unlikely to significantly improve an associated sexual problem, but should make it more possible for the individual to get benefit from specific sexual therapy.

5.24 Is loss of libido often a secondary effect of anxiety?

This is probably not so. Significant depressive illnesses, alcohol or drug dependence, or relationship problems are much more likely to be the key factor. It should be noted that sexual activity can be anxiety-relieving in some people as well as helping to promote sleep.

5.25 Is anxiety one of the commoner causes of insomnia?

Probably the commonest cause of initial insomnia, that is difficulty getting off to sleep, is anxiety and its related conditions. This difficulty tends to enhance sleep-lag, whereby patients find it hard to get to sleep, only get to sleep later, and then feel tired when they wake up. By contrast middle or late insomnia is more typically associated with a depressive illness. The syndrome of feeling 'tired all the time' probably derives in part from this early insomnia difficulty. Sleep hygiene approaches include maintaining physical activity during the day, avoiding excessive stimulants such as tea or coffee in the evenings, avoiding daytime naps, and having a relaxing routine, e.g. a hot bath prior to going to bed. While the median sleep time is about 7 hours, some people actually only need 5 or 6, and trying to sleep longer is probably not worth the effort.

5.26 Is anxiety associated with chronic low-grade conditions like candidiasis, ME or chronic hay fever and/or catarrh?

There is no evidence that anxiety causes any of these conditions, but clearly persistent unpleasant physical symptoms will be complained of more amongst anxious or obsessional individuals. It is also important to differentiate symptoms, in that patients may feel that their mood state (e.g. depression or anxiety) is actually caused by 'candidiasis', as their form of explanation. This may reflect fears of an untreated or dangerous disease, leading to a psychological tendency to magnify every minor symptom or unusual bodily feeling. Cognitive approaches to dealing with catastrophic fears about symptoms can be very beneficial in those with such 'hypochondriacal' presentations.

5.27 Can you die from anxiety?

A core fear, particularly in those suffering from panic disorder, is that they are going to die. This feeling that one is dying is probably generated by the 'fight or flight' response, and leads to the vicious cycle of symptom, catastrophic interpretation thereof, and enhancement of the symptom. Particular fears are of a heart attack, asthma, or a stroke, while depersonalization in those who hyperventilate can lead to a very strange sense of unrealness. This can even be interpreted as some kind of out-of-body experience associated with dying. Clear explanations of the way these symptoms affect patients can be helpful, although may have to be repeated.

5.28 Is suicide or attempted suicide a common outcome of anxiety states?

There is obviously a clear association of completed suicide with formal depressive illness, as well as with alcohol or drug dependency, social isolation, increasing age and certain forms of personality disorder. A somewhat different process of 'attempted suicide' (also called 'parasuicide') is linked much more to social and personality factors, being commoner in younger women, of lower social background and more limited educational achievement. It is also strongly linked with alcohol and/or drug abuse, as well as relationship problems. Most patients with significant generalized anxiety disorder or panic syndrome do not indulge in such acts, but there is an increased rate of anxiety/depressive disorders, as well as drug and alcohol dependence, amongst parasuicides.

5.29 Is anxiety more common in unsuccessful people?

Anxiety and panic disorder certainly impair social abilities, making it more difficult to get to or cope with one's work for example. There seem to be higher rates of anxiety and depression in the lower social classes, associated with higher rates of alcohol ingestion and use of tobacco, while those who achieve dominant social roles often have a very confident and outgoing personality style. There is also evidence that 'work stress' is higher in less fulfilled, middle-grade, managers, but whether this is a primary or secondary effect is uncertain. Patients who complain of 'stress at work' should always be closely examined for a potential, underlying, anxiety or depressive disorder.

5.30 Are there any medical and/or iatrogenic risks from anxiety disorders?

Unfortunately there probably are. Given the wide range of physical and psychological symptoms with which people can present, and the wide range of specialists they will see, a number are at risk of unnecessary medications, unnecessary investigations, and even unnecessary treatments. Surgical operations for irritable bowel syndrome, or invasive investigations for potential heart or lung problems, and drugs such as aspirin or steroids with their potential side-effects, can create significant complications. The importance of all general physicians having a clear understanding of the typical presentations and symptoms of panic disorder, in particular, cannot be overstated.

5.31 What is meant by the term somatoform disorder?

This essentially describes a group of patients who constantly develop a range of physical symptoms, requiring investigation, across a range of organ systems. The pattern of constantly seeking treatments despite negative investigations persists over a number of years, and does seem linked to higher rates of depression in the family. Such somatoform disorders can be distinguished from the process of somatization, which simply describes the tendency to attribute psychological symptoms to a physical disorder, for whatever reason. Particular forms of somatoform disorder include hypochondriasis (a persistent preoccupation that one has a serious illness), dysmorphophobia (a persistent and inappropriate concern that one's body is deformed in some way) or somatoform pain disorder, in which chronic pain cannot be explained by any obvious lesion.

The formal category of 'somatization disorders' is often characterized by associated depressive and anxiety symptoms, not least because both physical and psychiatric symptoms tend to change constantly. Treatment approaches are based on harm limitation rather than cure, but such patients do of course tend to move from doctor to doctor.

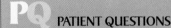 **PATIENT QUESTIONS**

5.32 Will my anxiety make me go mad in the end?

Anxiety symptoms are very frightening, by definition, and sufferers often think they will end up being taken into hospital and kept there. Because temporarily you feel out of control, dizzy or sick, and cannot think straight, it is a natural reaction to think things can only get worse. But the whole point about 'going mad' – that is, having a serious, 'psychotic', mental illness, like forms of schizophrenia – is that you do not think it is you that is ill. That is to say, as soon as you think or ask the question 'Am I going mad?', by definition you are not. And anxiety or panic states do *not* lead on to more serious illnesses, physical or mental – they may persist, or seem to get worse at times, but they are in themselves the problem.

5.33 Do doctors often make a mistake in diagnosing anxiety?

Half the problem of anxiety is worrying about having a severe illness that somehow the doctors have not got to the bottom of. If there is a problem, the doctors will often hunt around for some physical cause, even something quite obscure and rare, involving various blood tests or X-rays. This tends to make many people feel more worried, that somehow something has not been found, but the opposite is true. Thus, if you keep on having lots of unpleasant symptoms, like anxiety dreams, with all your tests being normal, that confirms absolutely the nature of your condition. Nowadays the types of anxiety disorder, for example panic syndrome, are very easily diagnosed and understood, and much more is known about their management.

Drug treatment of anxiety

6

6.1 Are there really any effective medications for chronic anxiety?

Yes, but there are problems with them being used on a chronic basis. Thus benzodiazepines such as diazepam, at a low dosage, 5 mg two to three times a day, can be effective for some individuals, even though there is a technical risk of developing tolerance. Likewise, continuing low-dose antidepressants, such as imipramine or amitriptyline (e.g. 25–50 mg – or even higher doses of 100–200 mg) show little evidence of long-term side-effects. The important thing is to monitor dosage, and adjust as required, particularly as people get older, and always to consider potential psychological interventions. Chronic anxiety is discomforting but not health-threatening, and is best dealt with by education, teaching relaxation techniques, and avoidance of stressors (e.g. excess caffeine, busy schedules). Judgements may have to be made as to upsetting the apple-cart in patients continually 'worried' but stable, and trying to force patients out of their (possibly cultural) limited social roles. The old Hippocratic saying 'first do no harm' comes to mind.

6.2 Are there effective medications for acute anxiety?

Table 6.1 lists drugs used in anxiety. Benzodiazepines, particularly those with a fast onset of action, such as lorazepam, are extremely effective and very simple to use. Every GP should carry oral and intramuscular (i.m.) preparations in an emergency bag, because acute anxiety reactions, whether in the home or at the road side after a crash, are very common. Depending on age and previous usage, 5–10 mg of diazepam orally, or 1–2 mg of lorazepam orally, or i.m. lorazepam 1–2 mg (even for psychotic illnesses) are standard treatments. Short-term usage, for several days, or for a week or two at most, while tapering off the dose, is also important so as to avoid the beginnings of tolerance or withdrawal effects. Clarifying the underlying diagnosis during this time will help with treatment afterwards, particularly if there is an on-going panic disorder. Introducing self-relaxation methods

TABLE 6.1 Drugs used in anxiety	
Benzodiazepines	Diazepam, lorazepam (brief/p.r.n. courses)
SSRIs	Citalopram, paroxetine, sertraline,* venlafaxine*
Tricyclics	Imipramine, clomipramine, amitriptyline
MAOIs	Phenelzine; tranylcypromine, moclobemide (reversible)
Others	Buspirone, propranolol, hypnotics (p.r.n.), mirtazapine
* Not formally licensed for use in anxiety disorders	

early, by demonstrating a technique or having an accessible psychologist, is also good management.

6.3   Why does medication so often seem ineffective?

> This is not surprising since even in the best-run trials, with their nicely cooperative patients, only 50–60% improve, while about a quarter tend to drop out, whether given medication or placebo. Since 'real' patients, as seen by GPs (rather than by researchers) are more likely to have co-morbid disorders like depression or alcohol abuse, difficult partners or fractious children, and variable compliance, these drug trial figures should probably be halved. The nature of the condition, in itself, makes it fluctuate in response to life situations, and the problems of misdiagnosis, sensitivity to side-effects and the difficulties of dosage all contribute to this. A systematic review of treatments, symptoms, social situation and patient attitudes can be worth the time spent doing it. Not taking the tablets – or stopping after one prescription – are much commoner than is recognized.

6.4   Are there any genuinely effective 'alternative' medications such as herbs?

There have been numerous trials, of varying quality, of homeopathy, drugs like St John's Wort, and a number of other substances. Looked at overall, doing better than placebo, which helps up to 30% or 40% of patients, is quite difficult, and there is no substantial proof for any one approach. Individual patients may swear by what they have received (e.g. from a 'herbalist' or complementary therapist), making them 'truly grateful', but as often as not they have responded to a longer consultation time, a sense of feeling listened to, and the active ingredient (for example in St John's Wort). Whether smoking cigarettes, drinking alcohol, or chewing khat or betel nut, people resort to a wide range of available, minor, anxiolytics, which is why for a low-grade, up-and-down, chronic anxiety state, psychological and relaxation approaches are always worth trying.

6.5   Is cannabis helpful for anxiety?

Cannabis is probably one of the most relaxing preparations – primarily owing to its active ingredient tetra-hydrocannabinol (THC) – and is available 'naturally'. Terms like 'mellow', 'laid-back', and 'chilling out', are integral to the culture of 'weed', 'spliff', 'dope', or what you will. In this respect it is like alcohol, certain cultural groups preferring to smoke a 'joint' – quaintly called a 'reefer' in the older literature – rather than turn to the sherry bottle. There is also some evidence that it can help some people with alcohol abuse reduce their consumption, while chronic use does lead to a sense of demotivation and mild memory problems. Patients who get unpleasant reactions, for example enhanced paranoia, usually are sensible enough to give it up quickly. Its possible effectiveness in chronic pain or dystonic conditions may well be associated with this anxiolytic property. There has, as yet, been no formal trial of cannabis in the treatment of panic disorders.

6.6 How addictive are benzodiazepines?

 The simple answer is that they are very addictive in those likely to become addicted. Anything that causes anxiety relief is powerfully reinforcing, because patients simply feel so much more comfortable, and wish they could be like that all the time. Whether one calls this euphoria, or an understandable human aspiration, the clinical problem is ensuring anxiety relief while avoiding tolerance or unpleasant withdrawal effects. Abuse is highly unlikely in patients without a history of drug or alcohol abuse, but the benzodiazepine withdrawal syndrome is very distressing. Depending on the patient, a withdrawal programme (*see Box 6.1*) may take up to a year, or

---

BOX 6.1 Benzodiazepine withdrawal

1. Agree outline plan and rationale with patient.
2. Agree on only one prescribing source.
3. Switch to equivalent dose of diazepam, nocte or twice daily at most.
4. Reduce diazepam by 1 mg to 2.5 mg per fortnight, or even per month if necessary.
5. Provide parallel relaxation training/anxiety management/CBT (whichever is available) and patient support group if possible.
6. If withdrawal symptoms develop, maintain current dosage for longer – use appropriate medications, e.g. SSRIs or MAOIs, if symptoms reflect returning illness.
7. Slow is better than quick. A year or two may be needed.

---

even longer, and will always need to be linked to encouraging psychological approaches, such as self-relaxation or even a course of cognitive therapy. Switching patients to diazepam equivalents (*see Table 6.2*), whatever their current benzodiazepine, is also good practice since dosages can be nicely and carefully adjusted down.

6.7 Is it safe to give benzodiazepines on a regular basis?

The fact of the matter is that benzodiazepines are very safe drugs, and while pharmacological tolerance is demonstrable, many people feel

TABLE 6.2 Benzodiazepine doses equivalent to diazepam 5 mg

Chlordiazepoxide	15 mg
Loprazolam	0.5–1 mg
Lorazepam	0.5 mg
Lormetazepam	0.5–1 mg
Nitrazepam*	5 mg
Oxazepam	15 mg
Temazepam	10 mg
Flunitrazepam (Rohypnol)*†	0.5–1 mg
Flurazepam (Dalmane)*†	15 mg

* Prolonged half-life creates hangover effect; repeat doses tend to be cumulative, especially in the elderly
† Not available for prescription via the NHS

psychologically stable without dose increases. While the guidelines and emphasis over the last 10 years have been to reduce consumption, this needs to be on an individual basis. Many patients are living positive, non-insomniac and relatively relaxed lives on say 5–10 mg of diazepam twice a day alongside a low-dose antidepressant, and why shouldn't they? Benzodiazepines are safe in overdosage, have minimal interactions with other drugs, and have no long-term physical problems associated with them, unless excessive, accumulating dosages are used, for example in elderly patients. While long-term benzodiazepine treatment should not be actively encouraged, it may be a least bad option for some chronically anxious patients.

6.8 Are antidepressants potentially addictive as well?

No. The core features of addiction, namely tolerance – increasing doses with less and less positive effect – and craving for more, are simply not part of the antidepressant profile. Nevertheless, research has shown that there is a strong public belief associating 'drugs' with addiction, and a tendency to muddle antidepressants with tranquillizers. This is not surprising, given their widespread use for anxiety relief, pain relief, and – in some people's eyes – relief of social difficulties. However, they do have withdrawal effects, which is not surprising since depression and anxiety tend to be chronic conditions that readily relapse. Deciding whether or not to discontinue antidepressants may involve lowering dosage and possibly thereby reawakening symptoms. Sudden stopping of medications should of course always be avoided, gradual discontinuation over several months being good practice. The short half-life of paroxetine, among the SSRIs, does seem to give it a greater likelihood of having a withdrawal effect, probably reflecting its greater, immediate, anxiety relief.

6.9   Which is the front-line treatment for anxiety today?

The benchmark is a combination of medication and psychological approaches. Every study has shown greater efficacy when these are combined, and greater durability when, in particular, cognitive behavioural treatment is involved. The current limited availability of this, at least within the British NHS, has tended to put the pressure in primary care back on to the use of medication. All patients diagnosed with an anxiety condition, whether generalized anxiety, panic attacks, social phobia or mixed anxiety/depression, require a full explanation of their symptoms. A standardized leaflet, as provided by the Royal College of Psychiatrists, and time spent in an anxiety management class, should be as routine as basic perinatal screening. Medication will depend on the patient's particular pattern of symptoms, physical health, age, and attitudes to 'drugs'.

6.10   What are the best treatments for panic attacks?

Treatments for panic attacks need to be considered in the short and long term. Benzodiazepines are the drug of choice, immediately giving good relief. They will not stop panic attacks recurring, however, and continuing treatment will require medication, ideally in combination with relaxation or cognitive behavioural therapy. Current first-line drugs would be either an SSRI (paroxetine and citalopram have the best literature base) or a tricyclic antidepressant such as imipramine, clomipramine or even amitriptyline. All will take time to work, need to be taken for at least 6 weeks, and probably 3 months to maximize their effect, and panic patients are very sensitive to side-effects. Using benzodiazepines as well for the first 2 or 3 weeks can help with this, and dosage needs to be increased slowly while monitoring the response.

Assuming no previous treatments – and it is always worth checking on what has been tried in the past – using an SSRI, then a tricyclic, and then a monoamine oxidase inhibitor (MAOI), probably the most effective but most difficult to use, would be a practical progression. Constant advice, education and clarification of the treatment programme, warning that it may take up to a year to get things right, is also essential (see Fig. 6.1).

6.11   Are SSRIs better than tricyclics in the treatment of anxiety or panic disorders?

Neither type of drug is more efficacious, but SSRIs seem to have fewer side-effects. Anxious patients are hypervigilant, and seem to magnify every little symptom, whether muscle tension, headache, a bowel movement or a heart flutter. Thus it is essential to use low doses first. That means 10–20 mg of

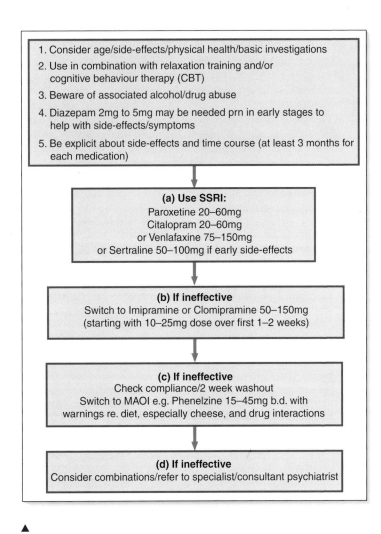

1. Consider age/side-effects/physical health/basic investigations
2. Use in combination with relaxation training and/or cognitive behaviour therapy (CBT)
3. Beware of associated alcohol/drug abuse
4. Diazepam 2mg to 5mg may be needed prn in early stages to help with side-effects/symptoms
5. Be explicit about side-effects and time course (at least 3 months for each medication)

(a) Use SSRI:
Paroxetine 20–60mg
Citalopram 20–60mg
or Venlafaxine 75–150mg
or Sertraline 50–100mg if early side-effects

(b) If ineffective
Switch to Imipramine or Clomipramine 50–150mg
(starting with 10–25mg dose over first 1–2 weeks)

(c) If ineffective
Check compliance/2 week washout
Switch to MAOI e.g. Phenelzine 15–45mg b.d. with
warnings re. diet, especially cheese, and drug interactions

(d) If ineffective
Consider combinations/refer to specialist/consultant psychiatrist

Fig. 6.1 Use of medications for anxiety/panic disorder.

paroxetine, citalopram or fluoxetine, 25–50 mg of sertraline, 37.5–75 mg of venlafaxine, etc. Tricyclics such as imipramine, clomipramine or amitriptyline should be started at doses of 10–25 mg, and only increased slowly. SSRIs are probably simpler to use, in terms of avoiding cardiac, overdose or sedation problems, whereas tricyclics will do better in those with bowel symptoms or previous bad reactions to SSRIs.

6.12 Are there any particular SSRIs that seem to be specifically indicated for anxiety or panic disorders?

Several of the SSRIs have obtained specific indications, in terms of their data sheet, for the management of these anxiety disorders, but studies seem to show that all are, essentially, equivalently efficacious. It is accepted that fluoxetine seems to have a tendency to make people more anxious or agitated for the first week or two, thus requiring additional benzodiazepines. This may be true for any of the SSRIs, but paroxetine and citalopram appear to have more of an in-built calming effect. Whatever the SSRI chosen, if enhanced anxiety or other side-effects limit its usefulness, it is always worth considering one of those two as an alternative before switching to a tricyclic or MAOI (*see Table 6.3*).

6.13 Is it rational or safe to combine SSRIs and tricyclics?

 Such combinations of drugs are best avoided, if at all possible, and specialist advice should be sought. They are used for the treatment of resistant depression, but their role in the management of anxiety or panic attacks remains uncertain. The likelihood of doubling the range of side-effects is high, and compliance with complex regimes – especially taking tablets two or three times a day – is known to be poor. To be rational one would have to use an SSRI only with tricyclics that have a primarily noradrenergic effect (i.e. imipramine, desipramine).

TABLE 6.3 SSRIs and related drugs in anxiety, depression and related conditions

Drug (brand name)	GAD	Panic	Depression	OCD	Social phobia
SSRIs					
Citalopram (Cipramil)	✓	✓	✓	?	✓?
Fluoxetine* (Prozac)			✓	✓	
Fluvoxamine (Faverin)			✓	✓	
Paroxetine (Seroxat)	✓	✓	✓	✓	✓
Sertraline (Lustral)		✓?	✓	✓?	
Other drugs affecting serotonin					
Mirtazapine (Zispin)	✓?	✓?	✓		
Nefazodone (Dutonin)			✓		
Venlafaxine (Efexor)	✓	✓?	✓	✓	

GAD, generalized anxiety disorder; OCD, obsessive–compulsive disorder
* Requires high dose – up to 60 mg

Nevertheless, if an individual feels 'better' by having an SSRI in the morning and a tricyclic, for example, in the evening to help with sleep and relaxation, that may be rational for that patient. Remember, combining either of these with an MAOI is extremely risky. Leave that to a consultant with a special interest in psychopharmacology, who is dealing with only the most resistant cases.

6.14 Is there any role for lithium in the treatment of anxiety?

The evidence for lithium is very thin. While being an established treatment for the prevention of relapse in patients with manic depressive (bipolar) disorders, acting as a mood stabilizer, and having some role as supplementation in antidepressant therapy (for resistant patients), it does not seem to be effective in the anxiety disorder, anxiety/depression spectrum of conditions. It has no obvious sedative effect, and can be problematic when used with some SSRIs. However, other mood stabilizers such as carbamazepine, sodium valproate, gabapentin and lamotrigine (newer anticonvulsants), do seem to benefit certain patients. These are well worth considering in refractory conditions, but more treatment trials are required at present, and again a specialist review should be obtained.

6.15 Are there any other medications, not having antidepressant activity, that can be helpful with anxiety?

The drug buspirone can be used in anxiety disorder, is not one of the benzodiazepines, and seems to be less sedating than them. In particular, it does not seem to have any addictive potential, but there is a lag in onset (several weeks) and there are conflicting studies as to how effective it is. Alternatively, the use of a beta-blocker such as propranolol can be helpful in those with specific, essentially physical, complications of anxiety, such as a tremor when faced with public speaking. This is best used on an 'as required' basis, rather than as continuing therapy. The use of non-benzodiazepine hypnotics such as zolidem or zopiclone, as a short-term treatment for insomnia, may also help at the beginnings of treatment if getting off to sleep is a problem.

6.16 What are the main problems associated with monoamine oxidase inhibitors (MAOIs)?

 Although originally used as antidepressants, the MAOIs are best established in terms of their treatment for anxiety and particularly panic disorder. The main dilemma is ensuring that a patient adheres to the diet, which means avoiding tyramine-rich foods liable to cause the 'cheese effect'. That is to say, hypertensive episodes occurring because the enzyme designed to eliminate monoamines has been fully or partially blocked. Such

---

BOX 6.2 Monoamine oxidase inhibitors: important potential dietary and drug interactions

Dietary*

Cheese

Bovril/Oxo/Marmite

Pickled herring

Broad bean pods

Food going 'off', e.g. offal/game/fish

Alcohol, especially Chianti/fortified wines

Drugs

Sympathomimetics (as in nasal decongestants)

Tricyclics (e.g. clomipramine) and SSRIs

Amfetamines

Fenfluramine

L-dopa/dopamine

Pethidine

Barbiturates

---

* An early warning symptom is a throbbing headache indicating a potential, severe, rise in blood pressure. The wide range of possible interactions means that practitioners should always check in the *British National Formulary* and warn patients as to what they eat and the risks of other medications (e.g. anaesthetics).

---

hypertensive crises can also derive from yeast extract (e.g. Marmite, Bovril), pickled foods, and stock cubes or packet soups (*see Box 6.2*).

The other core problem is the tendency for MAOIs to interact with every known drug in the book. Tricyclic antidepressants and over-the-counter cough and cold remedies are classic causes of difficulty, and most anaesthetists recommend discontinuation of MAOIs for at least a week if not longer before surgery. They are also dangerous in overdose. It is because MAOIs are such 'dirty' drugs, in terms of these interactions, that it is probably best to let initial treatment be managed by a consultant psychiatrist. The new 'reversible' MAOIs, such as moclobemide, may be safer but tend to be milder in their effects, though useful for anxiety without panic.

6.17 Is it safe to combine monoamine oxidase inhibitors (MAOIs) with other medications?

The simple answer is no, because of the many interactions that can occur between MAOIs and many other drugs in the *British National Formulary*. However, in rare cases of particularly resistant depression, the combination with tricyclics can be remarkably effective. It should be remembered that a drug-free interval, several weeks usually, is required before switching from an MAOI to another antidepressant, whether tricyclic or SSRI. The same principle applies vice versa, depending on the half-life of the particular drug. Seeking advice from one's local clinical pharmacologist or even senior pharmacist is always good practice in this regard. The combination of MAOIs with other antidepressants does not really have a specific role in the management of anxiety or panic disorder, but can help in resistant agitated depression.

6.18 How quickly will medication start to have an effect on anxiety symptoms?

The delay in the reduction of symptoms is a key problem, particularly in the context of panic disorder or social phobia, and more so if obsessive–compulsive features are associated. Benzodiazepines, of course, will immediately make one feel calmer, and thus can be useful for initiating therapy, alongside the other drugs. Studies of the effectiveness of SSRIs or tricyclics in the management of panic disorder show that they usually require at least 6–12 weeks of treatment, and patients should be advised of this at the outset. It is not the kind of onset associated with antidepressant efficacy (2–4 weeks), but a much longer-term process. Given this, explanation, monitoring compliance, and combining psychological approaches (e.g. relaxation training) are a vital part of the treatment plan.

6.19 Are there specific drugs indicated for specific subtypes of anxiety such as social phobia or obsessive–compulsive disorder (OCD)?

There is a strong literature, generated in particular by the competition between SSRI manufacturers to carve a niche for their own product and to establish specific medications. This has been done in terms of the use of high-dose fluoxetine, for example, for OCD and anorexia/bulimia, and for paroxetine in the treatment of social phobia. These medications certainly are relatively effective, of the order of 50–60% benefit in standardized trials, but the more these conditions are studied with other formulations, the more one realizes it is a class effect rather than a specific effect.

Nevertheless, it is probably worth starting with a product which has an agreed indication for that condition – and it also looks good if patients check up in their own copy of the *British National Formulary* or on the Internet – provided one keeps an open mind in terms of alternative treatment. The use of clomipramine, for example, with its strong serotonin reuptake-inhibiting effect, in the treatment of OCD, is very well-established.

6.20 How long should one persist with any particular medication?

Assuming there are no side-effects, the treatment of anxiety and panic disorders requires a long-term strategy. Building up to a full dosage for at least 2–3 months, particularly in panic disorder, is the bare minimum. Giving drugs for 2 or 3 weeks, at half doses, in anxious patients, is a recipe for enhanced anxiety, non-response, and an impaired doctor–patient relationship. The failure to continue with treatments – or to comply with them – for a long enough time is the commonest problem in the drug treatment of anxiety.

6.21 Is there any way of monitoring compliance or response to medication?

Compliance (some people prefer the term 'adherence') is a key problem for any medication, particularly for psychological conditions of some chronicity. At least 50% of tablets are simply not taken. Reasons vary from simple forgetfulness, ambivalence about taking drugs, and unpleasant side-effects, to the sheer practicalities of running out of medication and thinking that the course is naturally completed. Checking on compliance may be seen as intrusive, but can be done in a supportive way. Asking about side-effects (tricyclics always have some kind of side-effect, for example a dry mouth), checking containers, if the patient brings them, or asking for someone to keep a diary (e.g. +2 to −2 in terms of a self-rating anxiety or depression scale) can all help. Monitoring drug levels would be ideal, and can be done if necessary. Unfortunately the ranges are quite variable (in terms of therapeutic serum levels) and it can be an expensive business.

In the end, saying to the patient 'I don't mind if you haven't, but I need to know because otherwise I don't know if the treatment is working' – that is to say a therapeutic alliance – may be the only way.

6.22 Are there any specific withdrawal syndromes associated with drug treatments?

Just as with alcohol or opiate withdrawal, there is a very distinctive benzodiazepine withdrawal state in up to a third of patients if they discontinue the drug suddenly. Symptoms are those of a severe anxiety state, with a considerable physical component such as sweats, tremors, palpitations and insomnia. Even hallucinations and confusional states have been reported, and a similar condition is associated with sudden discontinuation of short-acting SSRIs, such as paroxetine. In fact, varying degrees of restlessness, difficulty getting off to sleep and depersonalization are commonly associated with any sudden withdrawal of a drug that is anxiolytic. Gradual discontinuation, over several months or more if need be, should be the rule.

6.23 Are medications effective in combination with psychological treatments?

There have been numerous studies showing that combined treatments, for example cognitive behavioural therapy with a tricyclic, or with an SSRI, is as good as or better than treatment with a single approach only. There is also evidence that the durability of treatment, that is a continuing remission in symptoms despite withdrawal of the treatment, is associated with psychological methods. By and large, therefore, if the resources are available, this should be the standard approach. Given the nature of anxiety, people's difficulties with somatizing, fears of having a more serious illness such as heart disease, and the stigma of being 'mad', explanation and reassurance on a regular basis are an absolute necessity. Furthermore, some patients will insist on something around 'counselling', while others hate the idea of 'talking treatments' and just simply want a pill to 'cure' them. Providing both should enhance the possibility of patients at least taking up one option.

6.24 How safe are anti-anxiety medications such as SSRIs or tricyclics if the patient is still drinking?

The combination of alcohol and any medication is an acknowledged problem, and patient leaflets usually suggest that alcohol should be avoided. The two major problems with alcohol are its tendency to block the effect of medications, especially SSRIs, and the possibility of medication enhancing the effects of alcohol. Thus, it is good practice to warn people that one glass of wine may have the effect of two or three, or might make them feel sick or dizzy, when they are on medication. By and large, though, these medications are relatively safe, and some patients may even find a reduction in craving for alcohol, if that is their problem. Clearly MAOIs and alcohol have a particular interaction (e.g. Chianti), and those prone to epileptic fits should be especially warned. If someone is abusing alcohol heavily, it is probably a waste of time, in reality, to try to 'cure' their depression or anxiety by going on prescribing antidepressants or tranquillizers.

6.25 Is there any indication for ECT in anxiety disorders?

If anything, generalized anxiety disorders and panics are a contraindication to using ECT. This is assuming there is no associated or underlying depressive illness, such as a severe agitated depression with obvious biological symptoms like weight loss, early-morning waking, marked self-blame and retardation. The main side-effect of ECT, namely short-term memory loss, will merely enhance the sense of anxiety that patients feel because of their difficulties in concentrating and 'remembering things', anyway. Part of the criticism of ECT has derived from its inappropriate usage in just these types of patients whose 'depression' was really anxiety or panic.

6.26 What is the role of beta-blockers in treating anxiety symptoms?

Beta-blockers such as propranolol have been used successfully for some patients with a very 'physical' type of anxiety. They are particularly good for those worried about some kind of public performance, for example playing an instrument or having to look calm and collected and not shake or sweat. By interrupting the vicious cycle of anxiety causing bodily symptoms, such as palpitations and tremor, they make it possible for anxiety-prone people to put on a good front as well as actually feel better. Chronic use of such drugs has been tried, even at extraordinarily high doses (e.g. up to a gram or more of propranolol a day) but there is no evidence of real benefit.

6.27 What are the commonest causes for drugs not being effective?

The common reasons for treatment failure are not actually taking the medication (non-compliance or non-adherence), not taking a sufficient dosage, or not taking it for long enough (*see Box 6.3*). Overcoming such reluctance in some patients is extremely difficult; thus the need for education and psychological approaches. Yet even in the best-designed studies between a third and a half of patients simply do not get significantly better, particularly if they have long-standing illnesses. Some patients really are resistant to treatment, others simply adapt to a sick role, and a few, let us be frank, are financially better off on benefits. But such patients are the exception that proves the rule, that it is not nice being chronically anxious. Most people appropriately seek treatments for their conditions. New medications, and/or combinations of medications, are still required.

BOX 6.3 Reasons for medication being ineffective

■ Non-compliance or irregular usage
■ Discontinuing medication too soon (i.e. <3 months)
■ Inappropriate dosage (usually *under*-dosage)
■ Side-effects outweighing benefits
■ Concomitant alcohol/illicit drug abuse
■ Wrong diagnosis, thus inappropriate medication (e.g. antidepressants for a paranoid psychosis)

6.28 Are anxious or panic patients at particular risk of suicide or self-harm with medications?

In terms of suicide, the key factors of increased risk are older age, social isolation, male gender, alcohol or drug abuse, depressive illnesses at the more severe end, and availability of method. Tricyclics should therefore be avoided in such individuals, if they are being treated for anxiety symptoms.

Use of benzodiazepines, antidepressants, and pain killers in deliberate self-harm – an overdose – are typical, often combined with alcohol. While anxiety may be a component of such patients' problems, formalized disorders such as social phobia or panic syndrome – or other formal psychiatric diagnoses – normally constitute less than 10% of such cases. Social problems, difficult and/or abusive upbringings, borderline characteristics, limited impulse control and drug/alcohol abuse are much more relevant in such presentations.

6.29 Is there any role for major tranquillizers in anxiety management?

Phenothiazines such as perphenazine or chlorpromazine have significantly anxiety-relieving effects, and can be helpful in those especially at risk of benzodiazepine dependence. They are also helpful in patients with paranoid or other quasi-psychotic symptoms (e.g. ideas of reference) and can even be useful in those with borderline personality disorder. This seems to be via a lowering of internal arousal, leading to less resort to self-harming events. Whether some of the newer 'atypical' antipsychotics such as olanzapine or quetiapine will be similarly useful, on a practical basis, remains to be seen. Their use is probably best confined to more difficult or resistant problems, and advice about side-effects and long-term usage is well worth obtaining early.

6.30 Does medication for anxiety as often as not have to be for life?

Usually not. By definition anxiety disorders tend to fluctuate, in terms of both frequency and severity of symptoms, according to personal stresses, time of life and random factors. If treatment has been effective using an SSRI, tricyclic or MAOI (and usually that will take 2 or 3 months anyway), it should be continued for at least another 3–6 months. After that it will be up to the individual patients, their personal circumstances, and their view of the illness.

Once 'well', many patients do not like risking becoming 'unwell', and keeping them on long-term, low/medium-dose medication is safe and effective. Others want to keep trying to become drug-free, so as to feel they are not 'ill', so gradual withdrawal, while being monitored closely, every year or two, is worth attempting. Between a third and half of patients will

not relapse again, at least within the next 2–5 years, particularly if given the
confidence of feeling they can deal with anxiety or panic attacks via self-
relaxation or cognitive methods.

6.31 Has the community psychiatric nurse (CPN) a role in medications for anxiety?

Recent regulatory adjustments have now made it possible for CPNs to
prescribe some medications. The standard antidepressants, whether SSRIs
or tricyclics, as well as minor tranquillizers, can come under this protocol.
Again, CPNs will need to take on extra training, in terms of understanding
the uses of specific psychiatric medications, but this kind of nurse
specialism is just what the NHS needs. Whether managing anxiety or
depression, however, CPN-led mood clinics are now well-established in
several centres.

 PATIENT QUESTIONS

6.32 I'm scared to take my medicine – can it hurt me? Is it addictive?

The cruel twist to being ill with anxiety is that it makes you frightened of
anything and everything. In particular, any change or upset in a safe routine
can easily bring on a panic attack, or the worry that you are going to start
getting a panic attack. In this sense an anxious person is like a nervous
climber clinging to a rock, too scared to move because he might slip. But of
course, if he does not move, he will have to go on clinging to the rock and
feeling frightened.

Taking medication – or embarking on any new treatment – is like this.
People worry especially about feeling sick or fainting, or becoming sleepy or
drowsy, so much so that they feel they will lose control. But this fear of
losing control is half the problem. The thing to remember is that all
medications have side-effects, but that they almost always disappear after
several days. What they mean is that the medication is having an effect.

It may take time for prolonged anxiety relief, or for panic attacks to go
away, but that probably means that the anxiety is being dealt with, not just
blocked out. Anyway, conditions that have been bothering one for a while –
months or years even – will always take time to respond. And remember, all
medications are very, very safe, many having been used for several decades.
They are safer than a number of over-the-counter drugs, like aspirin,
paracetamol or even some antihistamines.

As for fears of addiction, these are also very common and very
understandable. Not least because some people become anxious again when
they stop their treatment, and this leads on to feeling shaky, and getting
what even looks like a withdrawal state. Unfortunately these are usually signs
of the illness coming back again, although stopping medication slowly, step

by step, should always be the cardinal rule. Real addictive drugs – like alcohol, nicotine or heroin – are addictive because you want more and more to get the effect. Also they dominate your life, so you want to take them all the time, and they do not make you feel better. Effective treatment medications – as outlined in this chapter – work at a standard dose, and go on working at the right dose for you, and you only need to take them once or twice a day. Most people also start to feel better from them, so they find they can start doing other things rather than worry about medications.

6.33   The medicine isn't helping. What can I do?

If your medication is not helping with anxiety then there is a lot that can be done. First of all, do you remember to take it regularly? Many people do not, but just missing out one or two doses a week can halve the effect, which needs to be consistent. You also need to be taking the right dosage, as high a one as possible that does not give you bad side-effects, for a good 2 or 3 months. Furthermore, if one type of medication does not help, go back to your doctor or specialist and see if you can start on another one. All the time of course you can be reading up on self-management, for example relaxation techniques, listening to an anxiety tape, or attending a local volunteers' group. Attending specialized counselling, anxiety-management groups, or cognitive behavioural or behavioural therapy is also available, and such treatments can be carried out at the same time as you are taking medication. The two do not clash with each other.

If your anxiety has really been going on for a number of years, continually or on and off, then it may be worthwhile trying to write down exactly what treatments you have had and what you have not had, so as to have a really useful chat with the doctor. Although your case records will have a detailed summary in them, taking stock of all that has been done, what has helped and what has not helped, can often show the way to finding the right treatment for you.

Non-drug treatment of anxiety

7.1 Are psychological treatments effective for anxiety management?

If there is one area of psychiatric illness that does seem to respond to psychological approaches it is anxiety, in its various forms. The types of psychological therapy used in anxiety management are described in *Table 7.1*. Studies show response rates are between 60% and 80% in research

TABLE 7.1 Forms of psychological therapy in anxiety

No. of sessions	Therapy	Description
Various, by agreement 6 – open ended	'Counselling'	Usually 1:1; exploring feelings and background to current life situation, using reassurance and explanation of symptoms depending on counsellor's expertise
Usually 10–15	Anxiety management	Practical instruction, using group format, of the nature of anxiety and its symptoms; training in breathing control and/or self-relaxation
Usually 10–20	Behavioural therapy	Based on exposure (to the feared object/situation), with desensitization and measured assessment of anxiety relief
Usually 10–20	Cognitive behavioural therapy	Teaching individuals to recognize automatic thoughts that enhance anxiety and to develop alternative cognitions that are monitored (e.g. via a diary) and tested practically
Up to 3 years on a weekly basis at least	Psychoanalytic psychotherapy	Long-term technique aimed at exploring one's childhood and interpersonal style in terms of unconscious feelings (possibly repressed) that may be generating anxiety and/or depression
Usually limited to10–12 at most	Marital/family therapy	Aimed at clarifying one's personal relationships so as to involve the partner/family in resolving conflicts/stress factors

populations (i.e. in quite compliant and thoughtful people), so the clinical response rate may be less. Nevertheless, the basis of all approaches to anxiety, and there are successful outcomes, does rely on helping people understand the nature of their symptoms. Whether this is done via simple education, a formalized anxiety/relaxation programme, or via the use of books, tapes, or pamphlets, depends on the patient's needs. It must be stressed that while psychological treatments may not always abolish the anxiety, they do usually have an impact on unpleasant symptoms, and reduce their frequency, and make it possible for patients to deal with symptoms even when they do occur.

7.2   What is meant by relaxation therapy?

This is a simple technique (see below) that can be introduced in the surgery, and which patients can practise at home. It involves taking out set time to 'work at' relaxation, and also enables people to understand the relationship between symptoms, such as muscle tension, and how their body works. Individuals can work out their own pattern of practice or can use a tape, and a number of 'alternative therapies' operate on this principle (i.e. yoga, aromatherapy).

In the surgery, patients should be asked to sit, or even lie, in a relaxed position (*Fig. 7.1*). Just as if one were lining them up for a lumbar puncture, every aspect of how patients sit and how they lie should be closely assessed, so they are feeling as comfortable as possible. Having done this, they should be asked to tense up the forearm muscles for 5–10 seconds, then relax them, and then do the same with the upper arm muscles. They should breathe in when tensing muscles, and slowly breathe out when relaxing. Muscle groups in the abdomen, upper and lower legs, should each in turn be tensed and then relaxed, and the patients asked to concentrate entirely on doing this, emptying their minds of other thoughts or feelings. They should then be instructed to carry out a similar procedure, in a particular quiet place at home, with no one interrupting, for some 5 or 10 minutes, several times a day. They should also be encouraged to adopt just such an approach if they start to feel anxious or panicky in given situations, concentrating entirely on tensing and relaxing their bodily musculature. This process of distraction helps break the cycle of increasing fear and more pronounced symptoms, and makes it easier to get through the few minutes of a typical panic attack.

7.3   Is counselling effective for anxiety or panic?

Counselling may be much in demand, but there is no evidence that it reduces anxiety symptoms, reduces the frequency of panic attacks, or helps with understanding the nature of the condition. Of course, the term

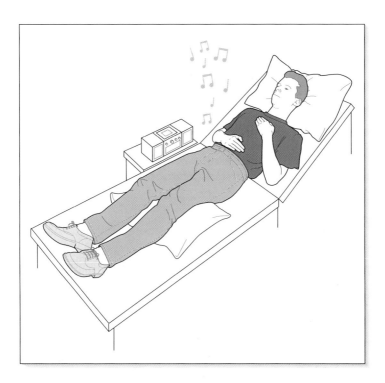

▲

Fig. 7.1 Suitable arrangement for relaxation therapy.

'counselling' can cover a range of approaches, depending on the counsellor's training. Unfortunately, this is not standardized, and while the ability to talk through one's problems can be of some relief, particularly if the counsellor has local knowledge of the social environment, it is not a treatment for an illness. Standard referrals to counselling, for people with poorly clarified conditions, can even be harmful. Searching for the meaning behind one's anxiety or panic in terms of one's childhood or upbringing simply does not help with the symptoms. Unless these are actively addressed, via cognitive or behavioural techniques, the patient will often just get demoralized.

7.4 Are there any particular self-help books or organizations?

There are a wide range of books and organizations (e.g. the Phobics Society) that can provide good-quality help. Trials are currently being undertaken of a computerized resource, and a list of potential resources, both written and on the Internet, can be found in the list of further reading (*p. 159*) and in *Appendix 2*. There is also likely to be a local self-help organization, possibly patient-led, and contacting one's local branch of Mind (the patient-led mental health charity), library or community centre can be very useful.

7.5 What is meant by behaviour therapy?

This approach to treatment is based upon an acceptance that behaviour is understandable, learned, and not necessarily related to deeper concerns requiring complex formulations. Thus, the tendency to have panic attacks in a crowded place is seen as reinforced by social stimuli, just as Pavlov's dogs started salivating when they heard the bells of the local cathedral. Once someone has had a panic attack in the supermarket, the reoccurrence of the crowds, noise, and heat, for example, will lead to a learned pattern of behaviour, namely a panic attack.

Therapy involves gradual 'exposure' to the feared object, having patients stay in a situation while reinforcing anxiety management or other relaxation techniques, and 'desensitizing' them to the feared stimuli. Thus, the behaviour therapist will accompany patients on a bus, help them with relaxing and slow breathing when they panic, enable them to stay on the bus, and even get off the bus and let patients go on their own for a while. Patients will often also rate the level of their panic, and be able to note the declining scores as treatment progresses. It is thus practical, related to real-life events, and measurable. Some 10–20 sessions should be effective, although longer treatment programmes may be needed for more intractable conditions.

7.6 What is meant by cognitive behavioural therapy and is it more effective than just behaviour therapy?

Cognitive behavioural therapy (CBT) is essentially an extension of the behavioural approach (*see Table 7.2*). Instead of the therapist instructing patients in, for example, relaxation, patient and therapist work together to look at patterns of thinking. Thus, a patient feels palpitations, and automatically starts to think of something catastrophic, like a heart attack. The vicious cycle of symptom and way of thinking leads to additional symptoms, and thus to a full-blown episode of panic. The cognitive therapist will help the patient develop an alternative pattern of thinking. Thus the therapist will try to obtain from the patient another explanation for the palpitations, for example 'I just had a cup of coffee', or 'This is just a normal variation', or 'I'm a bit stressed, but it will go away'. Patients will often be asked to keep a diary, writing down these alternative thoughts

---

TABLE 7.2 The cognitive behavioural framework

Typical problems	Increased anxiety; panic attack(s), i.e. crowded shops; increasing fear of social contacts, e.g. work/pastimes/travel
Thinking patterns	Fears are magnified and expectations of further panic become ingrained/automatic: 'I won't go there because I'm bound to have a "turn" or feel funny'
Emotional state	Increased worrying and fear of going out, with arousal and physical symptoms (feeling hot, sweaty, etc.)
Behaviour	Avoidance, such that people keep away from things they fear, leading to reduced social contact, rejection of friends, and acceptance of disability/limitations
Treatment approach	Identify, with patients, their ways of thinking, what their symptoms are and how they cope with them. Begin the process of suggesting/encouraging different thoughts/expectations, using a diary at home to record episodes of panic, precipitating factors and how they reacted. Encourage new thinking patterns and self-relaxation techniques that minimize the impact of further panic/anxiety

---

whenever they get an automatic thought about something awful that may happen.

Provided patients can grasp the process – of how they misinterpret their symptoms or feelings – this usually starts to show some benefit in terms of anxiety scores in the first one or two sessions. Depending on the condition treated, it can be equally as, or even more, effective than behaviour therapy, not least because it involves patients taking the lead in rearranging their automatic pattern of thinking (cognitions). Both approaches, CBT and behaviour therapy, do require the patient's cooperation, and that can be the main drawback. Getting the patient to attend the first session is often half the battle.

7.7 Can community psychiatric nurses (CPNs) train as behavioural or cognitive behavioural therapists?

Therapists usually come from a training in psychology and clinical psychology, but more and more are from a nursing background. This is because the key to such work is having a clinical grounding in the nature of anxiety disorders, and with specific training (e.g. as a nurse therapist) one can look after a whole clientele virtually by oneself. While behaviour therapy still seems best for simple phobias (e.g. fear of spiders), CBT seems more generalized, and thus more useful in helping other anxiety and panic disorders, as well as depressive illness. CPNs in terms of their own training and experience are ideally suited to develop anxiety management or cognitive behavioural approaches, which can be provided via home visits, in the GP surgery, or in day centres. In fact such skills should be part of the normal expertise of the modern CPN. The increasing demand for primary care mental health services, as reflected in the National Service Framework (and NHS Plan), will rely on community psychiatric nurses to deliver a range of psychological treatments.

7.8 Is it very difficult for CPNs to be trained in anxiety management or CBT?

Not necessarily. The knowledge and skills behind such approaches are essentially a refinement of basic mental health training. There is a bit more detail to be acquired about the physiology and psychology behind anxiety/panic symptoms, and one needs to become familiar with standard assessment schedules and the relevant distraction and relaxation techniques available, but these are not rocket science, and become easier and simpler to use the more experience one obtains. It's like driving a car. Once you've got the knack it is second nature to change gear while steering and checking the traffic.

As part of Continuing Professional Development nurses can also do recognized modules at their local university. Anxiety management tends to be incorporated within other areas, for example a Rehabilitation module would include 'management of a change environment', requiring skills in alleviating patients' anxieties. Half-day or day release courses, in association with clinical work alongside experienced practitioners, is probably the best approach. Effective CBT training can even be developed via intensive 2 week programmes, with continuing review of skills and cases subsequently. The Thorne courses are particularly useful (although tending to focus on psychosis), and nurses should not be put off by fears of complex theories and long-winded explanations. CBT is essentially a practical technique, not something requiring a philosophy doctorate.

7.9 Is there any difference between cognitive behavioural therapy given by a psychiatrist as opposed to a properly trained nurse or psychologist?

Essentially the answer is no, assuming the training for the nurse or psychologist is appropriate. CBT courses are well standardized, use a range of simple-to-use measures, and work via the development of alternative hypotheses, to deal with specific symptoms such as panic. A psychiatrist of course can provide a broader overview, in terms of using CBT alongside medication, diagnostic understanding, and dealing with more complex conditions. A nurse, however, may be able to relate more easily to a patient, will certainly be able to spend more time in tailoring sessions individually, and can work *in addition* to psychiatric treatments.

7.10 What are the standard rating scales used to assess cognitive behavioural techniques?

There are a wide range of these, usually used in research protocols, but few of them are practical for the GP surgery. Nevertheless the Beck Anxiety Inventory (BAI) and the Hospital Anxiety and Depression Scale (HADS) (*see Appendix 1*) are widely used, and are not particularly difficult to administer. The use of such scales can greatly enhance one's diagnostic confidence, as well as provide a means of clarifying to the patient the nature of the diagnosis.

7.11 How long does a typical course of cognitive behavioural therapy last?

The courses vary from half a dozen sessions to up to 20. This would depend on the level of the patient's response, in terms of measures of improvement after each session, as well as the patient's ability to grasp the process and the severity of the condition. The whole basis of CBT is that it is essentially practical, and can be carried out in any locality, by trained therapists. Good response in the first session or two is predictive of subsequent good response, while more than the usual 15–20 sessions does not bring much additional benefit (although the patient might welcome continuing to be seen).

7.12 Can such therapy (e.g. CBT) take place in a GP surgery?

This is certainly possible, and is the basis for the Government's commitment to add more psychologists to primary care via the National Service Framework and NHS Plan (*see Q. 1.23*). No specialized equipment is required, many patients may prefer being seen in the GP's surgery rather than a 'mental hospital', and regular follow-up meetings can be arranged. The effectiveness of a CBT-trained psychologist, or nurse, as compared to a standard 'counsellor' has been established in terms of formal research. The potential effectiveness of what CBT can offer, in practical terms, for specific conditions, is only going to be limited by resource constraints.

7.13 Are there any other forms of specific therapy effective for anxiety?

Other forms used include relaxation therapy, problem solving and solution-focused therapy. Relaxation therapy has been outlined above (*Q. 7.2*) while problem solving and solution-focused therapy are specific approaches that again are not difficult to understand. The former involves helping patients clarify what their real problems are, whether physical, social or a combination thereof, and by so doing encouraging practical ways in which each can be helped or even resolved. It is essentially a structured form of asking questions of people, and can help prioritize, and establish a sense of self-control, although it is no magic solution.

Solution-focused therapy, by contrast, looks at current resources and future hopes rather than present problems, and generally only uses up to half a dozen sessions. In this sense it can be usefully undertaken alongside other approaches. Getting the patient to see the solution is the essence of the approach, while also looking at what patients may already be doing, or trying to do, to help get to the solution. It is essentially based upon finding out people's strengths (rather than weaknesses, symptoms, and problems) and getting them to work on those. Just getting them to know, and clarify to themselves, what they would like their future to be (for example having no anxiety) in itself seems to clear some people's minds.

7.14 Can exercise be beneficial?

There is no doubt that exercise can be beneficial for both anxiety and depression. Regular aerobics, swimming, or cycling, which burns off energy yet maintains a regular rhythm, can help people understand how their bodies work. Exercise also helps with sleep – and difficulty getting off to sleep is a very typical anxiety problem – and improved sleep in itself leads to improved concentration, and energy and a sense of physical relaxation. The vicious pattern of tiredness associated with anxiety is very much related to this combination of unfitness, little physical activity, impaired sleep, and the sense of 'stress' one feels when tired and on edge.

7.15 What alternative treatments are available?

There are now some 50 000 complementary therapists in the UK compared to about 36 000 GPs, and over 5 million consultations. Up to half of those patients consulting GPs *and* psychiatric services for anxiety-related conditions have consulted a complementary therapist. While there are continuing debates about the effectiveness of such approaches, individuals often report feeling helped. Sessions usually have to be paid for, about £20–50 per session, lasting between 1–2 hours, and properly trained and qualified therapists will take a careful history, will not interfere with medical treatments and do offer time, attention, concern and an individualized approach. Some of the more popular therapies are outlined in *Table 7.3*, the treatment of chronic pain (e.g. back pain, headaches), bowel problems, and depression/anxiety/stress being very much the core of their work.

TABLE 7.3 Alternative treatments for anxiety

Cranial–sacral therapy	Specific form of touching/massage aimed at righting imbalances in posture and function
Hypnotherapy	Detailed discussion of history, then encouragement to relax, listen to the therapist and try to empty the mind of thoughts, imagining a state/scenario of total calm
Reflexology	Based on formal foot massaging with advice on nutrition and relaxation
Reiki (universal life energy)	Placing of hands on parts of the body in the context of a relaxed, scented atmosphere (including music)
Lightbody healing	Personality assessment via numerology and specific charts, then laying on of hands while asking for responses
Acupuncture	Discussion of problems (especially pain), then needles placed in relevant areas of the body
Shiatsu	Firm but gentle massage aimed at 'redirecting' the body into a more comfortable alignment
Herbalism	Detailed lifestyle questionnaire leading to dietary advice and the prescription of a number of herbs (c. 3–6) to be taken regularly
Crystal healing	Assessment of emotional state/life stresses, then specific crystals (e.g. clear quartz for depression, since it is uplifting) are held over various parts of the body deemed to need working on
Homeopathy	Detailed history then prescription of various selected homeopathic remedies
Aromatherapy	Use of selected aromatic oils (you decide the scents you like) massaged into the skin

7.16 How effective are approaches like yoga or hypnotherapy?

These essentially operate in the same way as anxiety-management classes, providing both physical and psychological relaxation. Some people find them very much the treatment of choice, although there is little evidence-based detail to show their effectiveness compared with, for example, CBT or behaviour therapy. The fact is that some individuals find them very helpful, and patients should not be discouraged from attending them. Most therapists in these approaches work privately, however, and patients will have to be advised as to the likelihood of benefit. It is probably wisest to support their attending for one or two sessions, but not to go on unless they genuinely feel an improvement has occurred.

7.17 Is there any role for specific books, films or plays?

Apart from joke movies like *High Anxiety*, anxiety, agoraphobia and panic attacks have not figured that prominently in Hollywood's canon. While specific training videos have been produced, it is difficult to think of a film that genuinely portrays the nature of panic attacks and anxiety, without resorting to a Freudian psychotherapist or extraordinarily intelligent 'counsellor', whose actual treatment approach is never clarified. A number of films, however, have central characters chased, watched or threatened by evil pursuers – for example *The Fugitive* or *Three Days of the Condor* – and then provide excellent visual images of the nature of panic. Shy heroines, such as abound in Jane Austen, also provide excellent descriptions of anxious experiences. A list of self-help books is given in the further reading section (*p. 159*).

7.18 Can music or music therapy be helpful in the management of anxiety?

There is no evidence of this being formally effective, although non-specific effects, as with many other alternative therapies, may be helpful. There is some evidence that the right sort of music, in shops or public places, can be relaxing, and may even reduce levels of crime. The use of a pleasant musical background that makes one feel good and calm when carrying out relaxation exercises (*see Q. 7.2*) can also be beneficial.

7.19 Is there a role for art therapy?

There is no specific role for art therapy in treating the symptoms of anxiety, panic or social phobia. It is generally used in a more non-specific way, helping individuals explore their own personalities, and enabling a sense of creativity and achievement in those unable to articulate for themselves in terms of language or other forms of behaviour. Again, as a non-specific adjunct to enhancing relaxation, or as a means of building up individual confidence, it can be most helpful. Many patients simply enjoy it, and by encouraging participation in a non-threatening group activity it can certainly help those with social phobia.

7.20 Are there any particular forms of group or family therapy that can be effective?

Unless it employs a CBT or a behavioural approach, family therapy is not specifically indicated for anxiety disorders. In more specific variations, for example carer or support groups, Alcoholics Anonymous or Narcotics

Anonymous, a group approach can clearly enhance the ability to, for example, remain off alcohol. A family-orientated approach can also help clarify family attitudes to the symptoms – they may be reinforcing, for example – and help break down their fearful or even catastrophic assumptions about potential 'heart attacks' or 'strokes'. Such sessions can also have a useful educational input, helping the partner or family to understand symptoms and to encourage changing behaviours.

7.21 Is psychological therapy more effective and likely to last longer than drug treatment?

There is no evidence that psychological or drug therapy is more effective than the other. There is increasing evidence, however, that those who respond to psychological therapies, for example CBT, do seem to maintain the benefits for longer than if they just had medication. This remains to be assessed over the course of a longer period of time (5 years or more), but the skills acquired via CBT – understanding symptoms, distracting oneself, developing alternative thoughts – clearly can continue to be used long term. Drug treatments can alleviate symptoms, but do not usually abolish them entirely; thus the need for a more psychological approach in preventing relapse.

7.22 Can a GP train as a cognitive behavioural therapist?

Yes. In fact, GPs should be excellent cognitive behavioural therapists, given their understanding of physiology, the nature and symptoms of these illnesses, and the kind of patients they regularly see in their surgeries. Keeping CBT sessions separate from routine clinics will of course be necessary, but the training does not require any specific academic or manipulative skill. Given the pattern of modern illnesses, it is probably true to say that every practice should have a GP able to deliver all or part of a CBT programme.

7.23 Is it always worth trying psychological therapy before medication, or vice versa?

This will very much depend on the patient's previous experiences of treatment. Many newly diagnosed cases will be reluctant to take medication in the first instance, because of attitudes towards anxiety symptoms and other psychological problems. Imposing medication on a sceptical patient is a classic precursor to non-compliance. It is probably best to explain both approaches to patients, namely a CBT or behavioural input alongside the role of medication, because combined approaches have the best outcome. A number of patients will have received various forms of psychological therapy, such as counselling or other 'complementary' alternatives, prior to coming to the GP surgery. In such individuals it is probably best to use medication (if they will take it), while patients who have been through two or three antidepressants, of whatever sort, are likely to be disenchanted. Sometimes a contract will have to be negotiated, agreeing to provide psychological approaches to patients while refraining from medication, but suggesting that if things do not get better within a certain space of time a combination at least should be tried.

7.24 If someone has benefited from behavioural approaches, does that mean they should receive further treatment in the future for further relapse?

It is generally accepted, in the management of all anxiety and depressive illnesses, that response to treatment at time A predicts a better likelihood of response to treatment from the same approach at time B. Thus, if a course of behaviour therapy has got someone out of the house, but the panic attacks have returned for whatever reason, it is likely that that person will respond to behavioural therapy again. 'Booster' courses of CBT are regularly used, although there is no clear-cut research on their effectiveness. From the point of view of psychological therapies, if one approach has worked it is well worth repeating it, since it will fit very much with the patient's views of how he or she can get better.

7.25 Is there anything further to be done for the patient who has not got better from medication, psychological treatment or a combination thereof?

Unfortunately there are a number of patients who simply do not respond to any treatments, and the key problem here is preventing them becoming demoralized. Some will accept a sick role and continuing social disabilities, while others will seek alternative treatments, or a second opinion. If a patient has genuinely been to at least two courses of well-constructed psychotherapy (behavioural and/or CBT), and has taken the full range of effective drugs (benzodiazepines, SSRIs, tricyclics, MAOIs), without benefit, then it may be worth stopping all treatments. This 'clearing out' effect can do two things. It will help the patient and doctor establish just what is the extent of the on-going symptoms, and it will enable one to evaluate any new treatment approaches that are coming in. Approaches to managing the chronic patient are outlined in *Figure 7.2.*

A planned hospital admission may be required, but there is an urgent need for specialist beds that most health authorities are reluctant to fund. There

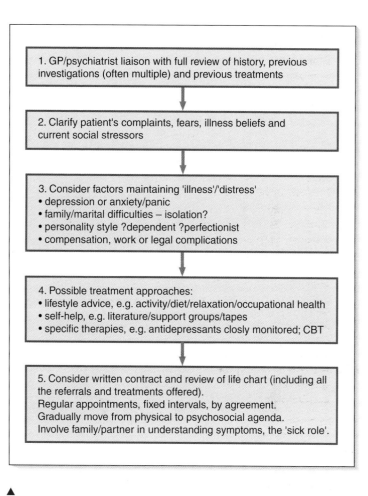

1. GP/psychiatrist liaison with full review of history, previous investigations (often multiple) and previous treatments

2. Clarify patient's complaints, fears, illness beliefs and current social stressors

3. Consider factors maintaining 'illness'/'distress'
• depression or anxiety/panic
• family/marital difficulties – isolation?
• personality style ?dependent ?perfectionist
• compensation, work or legal complications

4. Possible treatment approaches:
• lifestyle advice, e.g. activity/diet/relaxation/occupational health
• self-help, e.g. literature/support groups/tapes
• specific therapies, e.g. antidepressants closly monitored; CBT

5. Consider written contract and review of life chart (including all the referrals and treatments offered).
Regular appointments, fixed intervals, by agreement.
Gradually move from physical to psychosocial agenda.
Involve family/partner in understanding symptoms, the 'sick role'.

Fig. 7.2 Managing the chronic somatizing patient. (After Gill & Bass 1997)

used to be resources (e.g. psychosomatic units) that focused on these kinds of chronic, debilitating conditions – not unlike chronic fatigue or chronic pain states – but psychosis management now dominates mental health despite the greater prevalence of neuroses. However, the National Service Framework (NSF) Standard 5 does state that 'those requiring a period of care away from their home should have timely access to an *appropriate* [my emphasis] hospital bed, in the least restrictive place and as close to home as possible'. It will be up to local primary care trusts to push for just these 'appropriate' resources.

Although they may not be 'treatable', chronically anxious patients do need regular review, even if it is only every year or so (assuming one can keep them out of the surgery for that long), because new medications, resources, or other helpful processes (e.g. caffeine reduction) can come to light. However, some patients simply have to be left in peace, within their illness-imposed limitations, and providing sympathy and support can be more humane than simply tossing in another unpleasant drug.

PQ PATIENT QUESTIONS

7.26   The therapy I am having has not helped – what should I do?

The word 'therapy' tends to cover a range of approaches to psychiatric illness. It generally means a treatment given by a properly trained therapist – a psychologist, nurse therapist, or even community psychiatric nurse – that involves talking through your problems. Many people get referred to a 'therapist' or 'counsellor', who is happy to talk about personal problems – and this may be nice – but whose approach may not be right for anxiety symptoms or panic attacks. These may be related to aspects of your childhood, and it may be worth understanding why you feel so frightened in crowds, but stopping yourself feeling frightened requires a cognitive or behavioural approach.

Such approaches mean listing your symptoms, perhaps filling in some form of questionnaire, to evaluate how you feel before and after sessions, and perhaps doing some homework. This may involve keeping a diary, looking at where and when you panic, and what seems to bring it on. It may involve you taking certain first steps, for example travelling on a bus for one stop – at a quiet time, when it is not crowded – so as to build up your confidence for more demanding journeys. This would all depend on your symptoms and how you are responding to them.

Many people also require training in relaxation, so as to understand how anxiety works, how to calm themselves down (for example by deep-breathing exercises) and how to clear their minds of frightening thoughts. Again this will take training and practice, and will require you to think of panics as 'just anxiety', rather than as some kind of serious illness.

If you do not think your therapist, however nice, is actually helping with symptoms, then you should ask your GP to refer you to a specialist unit, such as the local department of psychiatry or psychology, that can undertake the right form of treatment.

7.27   Is yoga good for anxiety?

Most people would say it is. Yoga is essentially a form of self-relaxation, although a yoga teacher guides you in ways of calming yourself down. This will be by a combination of slow-breathing exercises, a calm group atmosphere, and adopting various body positions that you have to concentrate on. This not only stretches and relaxes muscles, but the sheer act of concentrating on doing things, holding positions, and slowing your body down, is often very therapeutic. Finding the kind of activity that makes you relax is the essence of managing your anxiety. Whether it is formal 'relaxation therapy' (Q. 7.2), or yoga, or aerobics, or forms of massage, does not really matter. They all help by working on your body and your mind, and it is worth exploring what is best.

7.28   How can anxious patients help anxious patients?

There are a number of voluntary organizations, the names varying from locality to locality, such as the 'National Phobics Society', or 'No Panic'. These can provide vital and accessible information, and patients themselves can act as a kind of communication pipeline to those who cannot for example even leave their homes.

Many forms of treatment, anyway, rely on the sharing of experiences, and this is particularly so in anxiety-management groups. These are based around a number of individuals, with similar symptoms – and all afraid they are 'mad' and not wanting to meet other 'mad' people – finding out that the persons seen across the room are suffering just like them, yet really completely normal inside. By learning tricks of self-relaxation, ways of preparing for potentially anxious situations, and that they are 'not freaks', patients benefit in a range of ways from such groups. They also, of course, learn to control their breathing, to relax themselves and to understand the real nature and meaning of panic/anxiety episodes.

A small group in my local area (East London) has established itself as HOPE (Help Overcome Panic Episodes), and such groups are very possible for people in all localities. Not everyone of course would get completely better, but the personal support, sense of not being alone, and understanding of the symptoms can all make life much more bearable.

The course and prognosis of anxiety disorders

8

8.1   Do anxiety disorders have a typical course?

The typical pattern is of relapse and remission, with a continuing vulnerability to enhanced symptoms in response to personal experiences, other illnesses, or a combination thereof (*see Table 8.1*). While patients who are just rather anxious, and have not had panic attacks, can often adapt by activity, dietary or lifestyle changes, those with panic disorder do tend either to get better or to retreat socially, into a long-standing agoraphobia. The longer either condition is untreated, the more likely it will persist despite treatment.

Strong family histories tend to reinforce and maintain symptoms, but increasing age often leads to adaptation. Preparing patients for longer-term treatment approaches, and trying different treatments intermittently can be of benefit. Because of this relapsing nature, patients should be advised of the real benefits of learning to deal with their symptoms, via relaxation training, cognitive behavioural therapy, or other methods as early in the illness as possible.

TABLE 8.1   The usual course of specific condition (*if untreated*)

Start	Condition	Course
Early adulthood	Generalized anxiety disorder	Chronic, fluctuating
Early adulthood	Panic disorder	Variable, fluctuating
Early adulthood	Agoraphobia	Chronic, fluctuating
Adolescence	Social phobia	Chronic social avoidance
Childhood/young adults	Specific phobia	Persistent (but often not socially impairing)
Childhood/early adult	Obsessive–compulsive disorder	Chronic, variable (esp. if *no* depression)
Traumatic event	Acute stress reaction	2–3 days
Traumatic event	Post-traumatic stress disorder*	3–12 months (usually)
Stressful life event (e.g. bereavement)	Adjustment disorder	Up to 6 months
Trauma/life events	Dissociative/conversion*	Weeks; up to 6 months
Early adulthood	Somatization disorder	Chronic/fluctuating

*Tend to be chronic if persisting for more than 1–2 years

8.2 Do people with panic attacks always have an underlying anxiety disorder?

Although they are named as two distinct conditions in standard classifications (for example *ICD-10*) it is most unusual for someone with panic attacks not to have an underlying state of enhanced anxiety. Whatever the basis of either, panic attacks can be seen as surges of unnecessary adrenaline in someone who tends to be over-aroused anyway. Of course, a few people with 'panic attacks' will be 'non-anxious' and may well therefore be having something else, such as obscure forms of epilepsy, genuine cardiac or respiratory conditions, or even hypoglycaemic episodes. These are rare exceptions that prove the rule that panic is actually best managed by lowering arousal, that is by anxiety management, psychological or psychopharmacological.

8.3 What is the usual age of onset for these conditions?

Typically people first notice symptoms, and report them to their GP, in their early 20s. A number will present earlier, for example in their late teens, and may well have a history of somatization (for example abdominal pain of unknown origin) prior to that. The question, to the patient or family, 'Has she/he always been a born worrier?', often hits the spot. Later-onset anxiety, for example in one's 40s or 50s, should alert the GP to checking out physical causes, but as often as not the anxiety in such cases will be part of another psychiatric disorder, especially depression.

8.4 Is there any typical starting event or experience?

Unfortunately no, although people tend to search for meaning. That is to say, they decide that a break-up of a relationship, a recent viral infection, or stress at work *must* be the cause. Distinguishing cause from effect, however, can be very difficult, especially in more chronic situations like work or relationships. Some people will describe their first panic attack, for example being stuck in a tube train, with great clarity, and of course panic attacks typically take place in crowded or closed-in areas, so it is worth asking about where it happened. There is also clear evidence that those who develop post-traumatic stress disorder (PTSD) symptoms usually have an underlying, anxiety-prone vulnerability, the trauma triggering what seems to be a latent state.

8.5 Can children be diagnosed with anxiety disorders?

A range of emotional disorders are described in children, including social phobia and agoraphobia, although these are not particularly common. The most typical is school phobia (to be distinguished from truancy; phobics being good in school, once they get there) in which a child becomes panicky about going to school, with associated anxiety symptoms. Sometimes it is mimicry of a parent's behaviour, and an agoraphobic parent will like to have a child at home to help out. Because of the different pattern of symptoms in children – as reflected by diagnoses such as emotional or conduct disorder – the diagnosis can be more easily missed. The prognosis for anxiety-prone and phobic children, by and large, is for significant anxiety problems in adult life. The effectiveness of treatment in preventing such a course remains uncertain at present, but should not be ignored.

8.6 Is the prognosis better for someone who has had anxiety after a specific event (e.g. a trauma) compared to someone who is a 'chronic worrier'?

As in all conditions, sudden onset has a better prognosis than a chronic or insidious onset, and this certainly applies to anxiety. Post-traumatic stress disorders generally only last for a few months, the images and flashbacks starting to fade as time goes by. In this sense, having a definite cause, or starting point, can be something of a relief to the patient. Likewise acute stress reactions, with an understandable basis such as an unexpected bereavement, should respond better to treatment. Positive and negative prognostic factors in anxiety disorders are listed in *Table 8.2*.

8.7 Do people grow out of it?

Yes, they probably do. Whether this is a genuine alleviation of symptoms, or individuals learning how to deal with them, is uncertain. There are few long-term studies and patients tend to be given a wide range of treatments.

TABLE 8.2 Prognostic factors in anxiety disorders

Positive	Negative
Relatively brief history (weeks)	Chronic state (years)
Clear stressor	No obvious cause
Stable personality (i.e. relationships; stable occupation; education)	Dependent/unstable personality (i.e. unemployed; poor schooling; unable to maintain relationships)
Good family background	Absent/dysfunctional family
Good intelligence	Learning/cognitive difficulties
Social support/friendships	Isolated/unsupported/ criticized
Insight into 'illness'	Abnormal illness beliefs
Early response to treatment	Poor response/non-compliance

Secondary problems, for example benzodiazepine or alcohol abuse, can also vary the outcome. When anxiety is associated with forms of personality disorder, for example borderline traits, clear improvements are only likely to emerge in middle age. There are of course a number of individuals who simply accept their disability, live rather constricted lives, but do not present as having continuing problems. This residual anxiety may only emerge in the context of later bereavements, early dementia or reactions to chronic illnesses.

8.8 Is there any association with particular forms of personality style or personality disorder?

There is a form of personality disorder entitled 'anxious avoidant' characterized by persistent feelings of apprehension, the belief in one's own social inadequacy, a preoccupation with criticism – and thus a restricted lifestyle – and a tendency to keep away from interpersonal contacts because of these fears of criticism or disapproval. In plainer language, this category summarizes people who are very shy. Other personality traits include people of the so-called 'borderline' type, characterized by mood swings, self-harm and chronic relationship difficulties. Those with tendencies to be histrionic and suggestible, or to be perfectionist and rigid, also tend to have secondary anxiety symptoms. Characteristics of these personality disorders – diagnostic descriptions that one should be careful of making too quickly – are outlined in *Table 8.3*.

8.9 Is response to treatment predictive of the subsequent course of the illness?

The briefer the illness, and the quicker the response to treatment, the better the prognosis. Patients who start feeling calmer within 2 or 3 weeks of medication, whether a tricyclic or an SSRI, are particularly lucky, since it is likely one can improve them and maintain them on relatively low doses. They are also likely to show better compliance. Likewise, significant change in the first session or two of a cognitive behavioural session is predictive of good outcome, and knowing this is important for clarifying the prognosis. By contrast, someone who has not responded to adequate doses of three separate medications, ideally of different classes, as well as a prolonged course of therapy from a reliable and experienced therapist is unlikely to get better from further treatment. Such non-response will leave people quite handicapped, and it is worth looking for maintaining factors, social or medical, in case anything has been missed.

8.10 How do people become 'heartsink' patients?

This term is not liked by many practitioners, since it seems to give a negative view of one's patients. However, it was coined because patients of

TABLE 8.3 **Characteristics of personality disorder/traits associated with chronic anxiety (from *ICD-10*)**

Dissocial ('psychopathic')	Irresponsible rule-breakers, low tolerance of frustration, thus readily aggressive and irritable especially if anxious/phobic
Borderline	Emotionally labile; unstable relationships and self-harming tendencies often associated with agitation, drug or alcohol misuse
Histrionic	Theatrical, labile, suggestible; wanting attention and excitement, thus overreactive to events/stress/hurt feelings
Anankastic	Doubting, perfectionist, rigid, wanting their own way and distressed/anxious when not complied with
Anxious (avoidant)	Persistent inner tension; low self-esteem; fearful of criticism, thus avoiding activities and/or social contact; easily anxious when rejected
Dependent	Indecision, subordinate, fearful of being alone and haunted by possible abandonment

All of these conditions are associated with a poorer prognosis when associated with significant anxiety/depressive symptoms

this type made one's heart sink when they walked into the surgery. In that sense it is idiosyncratic, different GPs generating different responses, and some GPs certainly having more heartsink patients than others. Research has shown that limitations in a GP's training and skill at interview are a key factor in developing or maintaining such patients. By and large, however, these patients, with their frequent attendances, wide range of symptoms both somatic and psychological, and non-response to treatment, are well known to most practices. There is evidence that identifying them clearly, and working with them, can, over a year or two, reduce their pattern of presentation (see also Somatization, *p. 81*).

8.11 Will our 'heartsink' patients always be with us?

When looked at over the course of time, heartsink patients do tend to either move on or gradually move out of the category. Direct action to identify them and work with them can be helpful, although not immediately. Attempts at reducing frequency of attendance can, however, lead to decompensation, and a well-structured, whole-practice policy – everyone has to play their part including receptionists and cleaners – is always worth trying. Recognizing the frustration, and honestly advising the patient about this, can also help with management.

8.12 Do social circumstances significantly affect the course of anxiety disorders?

Unfortunately the answer is yes, with higher rates of neuroses amongst those of lower social class in general. This is partly related to higher levels of single parent families and poorer living environments (e.g. noise, crime, unemployment, bad housing), as well as higher rates of nicotine, alcohol and drug use. Such social factors may even obscure the presentation, and such patients of course will use less sophisticated psychological language. They may also be more demanding for physical interventions or 'treatments' – an operation perhaps – for their problem, having a limited knowledge of – and considerable fears about – psychiatric approaches.

8.13 What is the relationship between anxiety disorder and borderline personality?

As outlined in *Table 8.3*, the borderline type of personality disorder includes emotional instability (mood swings), chronic feelings of inner emptiness, a pattern of on and off relationships and threats or acts of self-harm. Secondary alcohol or other drug abuse is not uncommon. The intensity of such patients' agitation can be quite frightening at times (e.g. head-banging), and they can readily generate panic responses – a kind of imposed sense of urgency – on those treating them. This constant pattern of crises is often the diagnostic pointer. Psychotherapeutically organized day hospitals are the best approach, although medication can be of benefit in stabilizing impulse control.

8.14 What about people who develop anxiety in their 40s and 50s?

Late-onset development of what is usually a condition that starts in one's 20s is always, by definition, worrying. It may reflect a form of agitated depression, thus it is important to seek out the depressive symptomatology underneath the mask of anxiety. Classic symptoms like early-morning waking, blaming oneself (rather than others), not being bothered to do the usual things, not even having a bath, and being unable to face the day (diurnal mood variation, worse in the morning) can easily be masked. The standard rule is that someone who has not been a regular attender, and who suddenly turns up with an odd pattern of symptoms, needs careful assessment including the usual blood tests.

8.15 What is the significance of the onset of anxiety symptoms in the elderly?

Elderly folk, psychologically speaking, are rather robust. The new onset of anxiety symptoms, therefore – and old notes should be checked to make sure it is not a recurrence – almost always means there is some significant illness underlying it. This may be physical, for example thyroid disorder or even Parkinson's disease, or an underlying depression. Given its prevalence, one needs to consider the beginnings of dementia, anxiety being the natural response to a failing memory or confusing experiences. A brief cognitive assessment – for example using the Mini-Mental State Examination (MMSE) – can be most helpful in clarifying matters. Older people's sensitivity to medications, whether for arthritis, heart disease, or psychological conditions, should also be closely reviewed.

8.16 Do patients with anxiety tend to change their symptoms over the years?

They are certainly a group of patients who seem to present a different facet of the neurotic spectrum of conditions as time goes by. Thus, presenting in their 20s with panic attacks, they will show obsessional symptoms in their 30s, depressive reactions in their 40s, etc. This may reflect a genuine truth, namely that our characterization of the different forms of anxiety is nothing more than the same condition presenting a different face depending on personality and social factors. The term 'cothymia' has even been coined to describe such mixed states (*Box 8.1*). Whatever the presentation, however, it is worth reviewing successful treatment in the past and returning to that. A 'booster' course of relaxation therapy, putting someone back on the tricyclics that got them well 10 years ago, or checking out their alcohol intake, may all be relevant.

8.17 Is anxiety really curable?

Anxiety symptoms can certainly be alleviated, but if someone has an anxiety-prone personality, or even a form of anxious/avoidant personality disorder, then that is what they are. In this sense, helping people to live with their tendency to anxiety will be crucial. Again, cognitive behavioural, or other forms of psychotherapeutic intervention, have a much greater

---

BOX 8.1 Cothymia: anxiety/depression as a single diagnosis? (Tyrer 2001)

- Common overlap of symptoms
- Partly inherited 'general neurotic syndrome'
- Similar modes of neurochemical function
- Medications (e.g. SSRIs, TCAs) effective for both
- Mixed anxiety/depression commoner than either disorder?
- Psychological approaches similarly effective (e.g. CBT)

likelihood of alleviating distress, even if this does not amount in fact to a 'cure'. There is also the consideration that patients are sensitive to other people's attitudes, and a cynical/sceptical GP can quietly but powerfully generate despair and non-compliance. The impact on other services, as patients seek help elsewhere, can be avoided by more active interventions. The NHS Plan, which aims to boost numbers of psychologists working in primary care, may really help in this regard (*see Q. 1.23*).

8.18 What are the key factors in deciding on prognosis in individual cases?

As with many psychiatric conditions, prognosis will depend on length of illness and the speed and completeness of response to treatment. The longer the condition, the less likely a response. Nevertheless, patients who are not drug or alcohol dependent, who have a supportive family, who can grasp the notions of psychological approaches, and who have relatively stable personality styles, will always do better. By contrast, someone with a chronic pattern of symptoms, a disrupted pattern of relationships and, for example, a declining work record, is not going to make a miracle recovery. Prognosis can be vital in particular when considering health insurance or reports for occupational health. Such chronic impairments should be considered actively for medical retirement (*see Table 8.3*).

8.19 If you are cured of one anxiety symptom, or specific phobia, will it by and large simply emerge as another symptom?

While anxiety does have a pattern of remission and recurrence, the fear that another phobia or symptom will emerge is probably unfounded. Good response to treatment means good response to treatment, particularly using the psychotherapeutic approaches outlined in *Chapter 7*.

8.20 If you have developed an anxiety reaction, such as PTSD, after an accident, are you more likely to develop one in the future if you have another accident?

Post-traumatic psychiatric disorders, such as PTSD, occur in about 10–15% of people who have experienced a frightening accident. Often this is a form of travel phobia, but can be more non-specific as a form of depression associated with pain, or relatively acute but brief, such as an acute stress reaction. Since those with a pre-existing anxiety proneness are in themselves more likely to have such conditions, they will be at greater risk of a recurrence. However, it is well known that people can have several accidents before, for example, a third leads on to a psychological disorder, while others can become inured to subsequent events. Those who have experienced unpleasant, post-accident, symptoms, should be advised to see their doctor as soon as possible if they have another accident, because early sedation and/or pain relief may significantly protect them from continuing disability.

8.21 Do individuals actually die from severe anxiety or panic states?

In themselves, anxiety and panic, although bringing on the fear of death, are not life-threatening. The problem is that the symptoms are biologically designed to create such inner arousal that you will flee or avoid the feared situation. The intensity of this experience will vary from patient to patient, and can lead to secondary risks. Thus someone with pre-existing heart disease may develop a dysrhythmia, and someone with severe obstructive lung disease may develop a severe asthmatic reaction. In this sense the anxiety has been a precursor to what may turn out to be a terminal heart attack, for example, but the pre-existing disease will have created the true vulnerability. A good analogy would be the known incidence of sudden heart attacks in otherwise fit men playing squash.

The importance of actively treating anxiety or panic attacks, in those with compromised lung or cardiac function, is obvious. Tailoring medication to their needs will usually require a specialist opinion. The only other risk is that of people panicking such that they jump out of cars or buses, or rush out of shops into a busy street. States of absolute terror, leading to defenestration (i.e. jumping out of high windows) or air rage, are almost always associated with alcohol abuse or withdrawal. Thus delirium tremens, for both physical and psychological reasons (mostly physical, it must be said), has about a 5–10% mortality.

8.22 Do some patients like being constantly ill and playing the 'sick role'?

Differentiating between chronic anxiety/depressive states, somatoform disorders, and malingering, is extremely difficult. As often as not it is a mixed picture, people with a persisting panic disorder finding themselves unable, for example, to cope with the journey in to work. They can do it, if really pushed, but the sheer relief of not having to go out because they are 'sick' deserves some sympathy. Disappointments in living, alongside persisting symptoms (whether pain, fatigue or panic attacks) can naturally lead to the status of disability being a safe harbour in which to shelter. A number of intractable, long-standing neurotic illnesses, whether anxiety, depression or obsessional, can so handicap individuals that this is a reasonable way of accepting their limitation.

However, the rules of the 'sick role' are that while accepting that the disease is unscheduled, involuntary and releases one from social duties (i.e. is time off) it is also accepted that the patient really wants to get well and will seek and comply with treatment. Thus when patients do not take their pills, seem to have other reasons for getting time off, and essentially do not play by the rules of being ill, it becomes most frustrating to a treating doctor. In such situations honesty and clarity are the best policy. Being absolutely clear about the diagnosis, the treatment plan and the likely outcome may require referral to a consultant, to reinforce matters. Likewise, not being sure about the diagnosis – and anxiety disorders can be quite difficult to characterize in some individuals, over the course of time – is part of the core problem underlying this collection of diseases. Such uncertainty will fuel a patient's fears of a 'serious' underlying illness, like cancer or heart disease, and specialist advice is therefore even more usefully sought.

8.23 Are there risks in treating vigorously someone who has had a chronic illness for many years?

There certainly are, because of the accepted range of disabilities that those with chronic illnesses have taken on. This may include regular benefits (e.g. Disability Living Allowance or its variants), a particular social role that demands some kind of care, and a pattern of activities that is limited by agreement. These are essentially social problems, however, rather than medical problems, and there are no real medical risks in making someone better from chronic panic attacks, for example. Clearly those who have not left the house for several years will be, to some degree, physically unfit, and a graded exercise programme might be necessary. One also needs to consider the carers, who might have unreasonable expectations of new, vigorous treatments, or even be put out by a newly 'healthy' relative. Being cautious about prognosis is an absolute rule in chronic conditions.

8.24 Are there any preventive strategies to reduce the risk of chronicity in those presenting with anxiety symptoms?

Prevention of mental illness remains something of a sore topic, given our limited knowledge of the real aetiology, apart from obvious factors like bereavement, life-threatening, 'traumatizing' events, such as car crashes, or the childhood environment. The most consistent factor associated with chronicity is a tendency to somatize, and to have had numerous assessments, investigations and half-treatments without any satisfactory outcome. An agreed protocol or guideline, for the initial assessment, management and continuing care of people who have essentially anxiety-based conditions – agreed with one's local community mental health team and/or consultant psychiatrist – should be a good way forwards. Involving a community psychiatric nurse (CPN) early in such assessments, by ensuring the ready availability of CPNs in primary care, may be the most useful practical step. The National Service Framework (NSF) does insist on this as a standard.

Of course, the problem with most guidelines is that they end up on the shelf; thus a regular liaison clinic, for example, with a consultant colleague can keep the memory fresh. An established anxiety management programme (nurses, OTs or psychologists leading it), where patients are educated about the symptoms they are having, given self-help strategies, and allowed to meet others with the same condition – thus seeing that they are not 'mad', a common fear – should also be of benefit. The possible need for continuing treatment, over several years, with an effective medication should also be discussed openly. As with depression, inadequate dosage for an inadequate period of time is the commonest reason for non-response when potentially useful medication is employed.

8.25 Can patients with chronic anxiety disorders get back to work?

This is an increasing dilemma for GPs, especially with the recent insistence on 'work stress' in some occupational health and legal circles. The fact of the matter is that many people can cope with work despite anxiety/depression, but it is often rather a subjective assessment. Use of standardized scales (e.g. HADS – *see* Q. 3.2) can help clarify matters. Factors that need consideration are outlined in *Box 8.2*. It should not be a GP's job to decide exactly if Mrs X is suitable for job Y – that is what occupational health specialists are paid to decide. The nature of the symptoms, their likely effect on core abilities (e.g. can the patient lift things, concentrate on a task like typing, deal with the public, cope with timetables and a structured day) and the background history of treatment and response/non-response are what one needs to outline. Continuing symptoms and worklessness for more than 2 years have a poor prognosis, whatever the diagnosis. Assuming several proper courses of treatment have been tried, without relief, then medical retirement is likely to be the most sensible option.

BOX 8.2 Advising on medical retirement for anxiety/depression disorders

Factors that need to be considered include:

- The length of the illness (>2 years continuous = poor outlook)
- The effect of particular symptoms on work performance (e.g. anxiety in social contacts ≡ social phobia)
- The occupational history:
  - ? always/usually in work
  - ? stability of employment
  - ? reasons for changing jobs
- The effects of treatment, over how long?
- Background personality style ± 'disorder'.

8.26 What is the prospect for new forms of treatment in the course of the next 10 years?

The increased availability, via training programmes, of cognitive behavioural therapy – using nurse practitioners as well as even a computer programme – is the most likely, genuine improvement that we will have in the next decade (*see Box 8.3*). Techniques and approaches are also being refined, in order to clarify what sort of patients can really benefit from such treatments, as well as how long treatments need to be employed. In terms of medication, our understanding of the neurochemistry behind enhanced anxiety is increasing, and we can expect more sophisticated GABA receptor agonists to be produced. We can also expect the development of 'smarter' SSRIs, a possible role for some of the newer anticonvulsants (e.g. gabapentin, lamotrigine), alone or in combination with standard treatments, and even the use of some dopamine-active agents. For example, atypical antipsychotics, with mild dopamine-blocking activity as well as serotonin activity, may be helpful given recent brain studies showing the role of dopamine in social phobia. Whether taking a psychological or pharmacological approach, the importance of combination treatments is increasingly being recognized, and we can expect some established combinations to emerge.

Even with the most modern of medications, however, little progress will be made unless patients are properly diagnosed. Aids such as computer-based diagnosis, good-quality questionnaires and/or standard checklists, and specific training programmes – for example via the revalidation and continuing professional development (CPD) programme – should also help enormously.

BOX 8.3 New approaches to anxiety disorders

1. *Prevention* – via health promotion; schools projects, anti-stigma campaign; dietary advice (e.g. caffeine, alcohol)
2. *Assessment* – computerized interviews; TV educational/interactive programmes; primary care mood clinics
3. *Treatment* – cognitive and anxiety management techniques used by CPNs; innovative medications acting on GABA system; collaborative care combining psychological and pharmacological interventions by a specialist team (Roy-Byrne at al 2001).

PQ PATIENT QUESTIONS

8.27 I had been feeling well for years and thought I was free of anxiety. Now it has started again. Why?

Anxiety, and the various physical and psychological symptoms that go with it, are part of the normal reaction to a whole range of problems. These may be physical – a bad dose of flu or a painful injury – or more psychological, like pressure at work or relationship difficulties. If you are something of a born worrier then that will be your response to these stresses, although sometimes there is no actual stress at all. In this sense the tendency to have an anxiety attack is always there, waiting to be stirred up, just like someone with pale skin getting painfully sunburnt on a hot day.

The trick is to go back to doing the things that got you better before. This may involve practising relaxation, changing diet or activities, or even taking medication again for a while. Since your anxiety has gone away before, the chances are high that it will go away again, even if there is no obvious cause for it coming on. In this sense anxiety illnesses do tend to come and go naturally, for reasons that are unclear; and this is a most important point to keep in mind, as a 'non-catastrophic' thought. Just realizing that anxiety does come and go, like the seasons, and getting on with doing the right things can in themselves help start you feeling better.

8.28 Do I have to live with this problem for the rest of my life?

Probably not. If you are prone to anxiety, to being a 'worrier', then you are likely to have times when you do get anxious, or even panicky, on and off. The interesting thing about anxiety is that it becomes less of a problem as you get older, so people do, really, 'mellow out' with time. This applies not just to anxiety, but to the kind of depressions that often go with anxiety, and the on/off physical symptoms (like palpitations) that go with them. It is also probably true that most people do find some kind of treatment that works, whether medication or psychological or whatever, and adapt their lives so as to avoid the anxiety interfering too much in their day-to-day activities.

Case histories

9

Case vignettes are a helpful and practical way of illustrating the personal and clinical essentials of typical presentations. Given the distinct nature of many, but certainly not all, of the forms of anxiety disorder, a pattern of quite 'typical' stories does emerge. Summarized below are seven cases, aimed at illustrating the essentials of the relevant conditions. They are based on an amalgam of outpatient assessments over the last few years, and have been carefully anonymized. If any one case seems recognizable, in whole or in part, that should not be surprising, because common conditions occur commonly, and there is a common pattern of symptoms that should enhance clinical confidence in diagnosis.

9.1 A typical case of panic syndrome, or depression?

Mrs B was a 37-year-old woman, referred by her GP with a history of being 'depressed for about 2 years'. She was prescribed an SSRI, which she took intermittently for several months, with no benefit. When asked about what *she* meant by 'depression' she actually described increasing anxiety feelings in closed-in spaces, going back for some 5 years. She gave a particular example of feeling that she was 'trapped' on underground trains.

She also described episodes of feeling very hot and shaky, with a sense of the world closing in on her, leading to an urgent desire to get home as soon as possible. These had been occurring regularly for the last 2 years, with no obvious event setting them off. As a result she had preferred to stay indoors, and now needed her daughter to go with her in order to go shopping. She also described random changes of mood ('mood swings') when she became snappy and tearful.

Asked about any other physical symptoms, she felt her weight had gone up (along with her appetite) and at times she tended to binge eat. She mentioned waking sometimes (but not usually) at 4 in the morning, finding it hard to get back to sleep. She often felt worse in the morning, finding it hard to concentrate then, and admitted to at times wanting to check things more than others would. For example, whether she had shut the door on leaving home, even though her daughter was with her.

Background history review showed no evidence of previous illnesses, medical or psychiatric. However, her childhood had been disrupted by parental arguments, and she had never done particularly well in school. Nevertheless she had a stable relationship, over 20 years, and two apparently 'sensible' teenage children. She did admit to drinking alcohol more heavily about a year previously, for about 6 months, but became worried about this, and rather argumentative, and thus managed to cut down. In terms of formal examination there was nothing of note, in that she was quite friendly and coherent, but a bit anxious. She had managed to get to the hospital on her own, because it was luckily nearby, but did admit that she hoped the interview would be over quickly. She seemed to have some insight into the fact that she had a problem, and was worried that it was just her being a bit silly and stupid about things.

When taken through her experiences of a panic attack, in terms of palpitations, sweats, feeling 'depersonalized', and feeling horribly self-conscious, it became clear that she had very typical symptoms. Asked about taking her medication, she admitted she had not really taken it very often, but was willing to give it another go. She was reluctant about possibly attending a 'group' – 'I feel embarrassed talking to strangers' – but she agreed to at least an assessment from the physiotherapist running a formal anxiety management group.

On follow-up 1 month later, however, she had missed the appointment, but admitted she was feeling a little bit sick from her medication and was switched to imipramine at a 10 mg nocte starting dose, with incremental increases over a month up to 50 mg at night. A month later she had managed to comply with this, agreed she was sleeping rather better, and had in fact managed to go out twice on her own. She was given the phone number of a voluntary organization, specializing in dealing with panic attacks, and subsequently made several contacts.

Although unable to tolerate a higher dose of imipramine than 50 mg, after 6 months she had settled into a pattern of feeling better in herself, going out intermittently but still being somewhat reliant on her family. Eventually she decided to move to a semi-rural location, and was lost to follow-up.

COMMENTS

This woman had a typical panic disorder with agoraphobia, that is to say inability to cope with crowded 'marketplace' situations, a temporary resort to an almost dependent usage of alcohol, which she solved herself, and some secondary depressive symptoms. She made a partial improvement with a combination of medications and anxiety management (albeit from a voluntary group rather than professionals), and ended up solving her difficulties to some degree by moving to a 'quieter' area. Her symptoms and social response are typical, and the prognosis would be for intermittent relapses, when confronted by difficulties (e.g. bereavements), but her insight is likely to enable her to take up extra treatment as required.

9.2   Is dysthymia really different from depression?

Mr B, a 32-year-old man with a history of 'depression' described by his general practitioner as having been 'semi-continuous since his teens', was referred for review having been on a low-dose tricyclic antidepressant for about a year without improvement. He had also been attending group counselling for about 5 years, but was continuing to experience troubling symptoms.

These included a general sense of 'feeling down', and finding it hard to get things done to completion. He described one or two apparently traumatizing events in his childhood, for example seeing his father slap his mother, and several hasty separations, associated with his father being very angry and hitting him. Nevertheless he reported his parents as still together, and no other formal family history of illness.

In terms of his daily routine, he described difficulties in getting off to sleep, occasional bad dreams, and sometimes waking early in the morning, but not always. He had a constant sense of not having enough energy, and sometimes feeling quite tired by day, for reasons he could not clarify. His appetite was limited, but he had not lost any weight, and he was able to do day-to-day tasks, for example cleaning or shopping when not too tired.

There was no previous medical or psychiatric history of note, but he admitted to being rather dependent on his wife (he had been married for 10 years) who was the breadwinner, working as a secretary. He had helped out intermittently with a family shop, but had not been able to develop any consistent career pattern. There were no children, but he reported his wife and himself as not being especially distressed by this. He was a regular smoker (about 15–20 a day) and worried that he might be drinking a bit more alcohol than in the past. This only amounted, however, to two or three glasses of wine at night on two or three days of the week, but he felt he had limited social contacts and, at times, tended to worry about his wife becoming bored with him.

In terms of his presentation, he was quite smartly dressed, neatly groomed, and not obviously slowed down or anxious. He described a sense of feeling low, subjectively, with no particular pattern of mood state during the day, and came across generally to the interviewer as someone who was somewhat sad and down at heart. He complained of some memory problems, but a cognitive assessment showed good levels of concentration and recent memory, and there was no evidence of other specific symptoms such as panic attacks, phobias, or *unusual* experiences (e.g. hallucinations).

COMMENTS

Given the background and rather long history, and the lack of any striking symptoms, a provisional diagnosis of dysthymia was made, based on the evidence of a chronic, low-grade depressive state, with associated lifestyle limitations. The lack of any more striking features (e.g. marked self-blame, retardation) also pointed to such a diagnosis, while the family history of a likely mood/alcohol disorder in the father was not untypical.

Given the limited impact of antidepressant therapy (he had been on SSRIs prior to his current tricyclics) it was felt best to refer him to a day hospital programme with a cognitive therapeutic approach. This involved individual and group activities, work looking at an alternative self-image to his somewhat depressive viewpoint, and referral to the gym (yes!) for some fitness work.

Follow-up a year later, from the GP, revealed a much lower attendance rate (only three times in the previous year), his enrolment in a computer course and his not being on any medication. He continued to complain of feeling 'depressed' but remarked to the GP, spontaneously, that he had decided to get on with his life nevertheless.

9.3 Is there a typical form of post-traumatic stress disorder?

Mrs C, a 38-year-old mother of two, was driving home one rainy evening on the motorway. She had her two small children (aged 5 and 7) in the back seat of the car, and it was raining. Pulling off on to a slip road she noticed with alarm another car coming against her which slammed into the offside of her car. She was thrown backwards and forwards and felt stunned, taking several minutes to recover her wits.

She then thought she noticed steam, or even smoke, coming out of the car, and she tried to get out. The door was jammed, her children were crying, and she became very frightened. After a few minutes the door was forced open by a workmen from a passing lorry, and she was able to get herself and her two small children out. She felt very wobbly, her neck was starting to become painful, and she was crying hysterically. After the usual delays she was taken to hospital with her children, given painkillers, and eventually reached home after midnight feeling tense and exhausted.

Over the next 2 weeks she slept badly because of neck pain, despite analgesics from her GP. She was thinking about the accident during the day, and found that it preyed on her mind. She could not get the thought out of her mind that she might have been killed, or her children killed, had the car gone up in flames. She began having nightmares, which woke her, felt tense and snappy by day, became withdrawn and rather distant from her husband, and found it very difficult to get back into a car. Driving would constantly remind her of images from the accident (e.g. screeching tyres or cars looming up fast beside her), she was finding it hard to get off to sleep, and finding it difficult to cope with day-to-day tasks.

Because of her tearfulness and tension the GP referred her for counselling, but after attending two sessions she did not feel it was being helpful. She was also prescribed sleeping tablets, and eventually (some 4 months after the accident) an SSRI. This made her feel a bit calmer, but did not abolish her nightmares, her travel anxiety or her tendency to run through the scenario in her mind. Eventually, however, things began to improve, such that by about 9 months after the accident she was only having the occasional nightmare, was sleeping better, was less snappy (by her husband's report) and felt she was no longer dominated by the accident.

There was no background history of note, she had some perfectionist traits but no evidence of previous anxiety symptoms, and she was a non-drinker. She continued to feel anxiety when driving – and was aware of how irritating she was as a passenger – but agreed to do an advanced driving course, which helped to some degree. By about a year after the accident her sleep, mood state and concentration were back to almost normal, she was coping better with her children, and it took very specific reminders to make her think of the accident any more.

COMMENTS

This woman suffered from a very typical post-traumatic state, with nightmares, 'flashbacks' (daytime visualizations of the accident), impaired sleep and concentration and a mixed pattern of anxiety/depressive symptoms. Neither counselling nor medication really helped much, but the passage of time led to gradual improvement. She was eventually awarded some compensation, which included something for a mild to moderate post-traumatic stress disorder (PTSD), agreed by the experts from both parties. She used it as part payment for a large 'solid' family car.

9.4 Generalized anxiety disorder – is there a typical case pattern?

Mrs M, a 25-year-old European immigrant, with no previous medical history of note, had had a number of symptoms since coming to the UK 3 years earlier. In particular she experienced headaches, impaired sleep, occasional difficulty breathing, and a sense of pressure round her head. She was thus taking Migraleve, diazepam and other painkillers in variable amounts, and had also been prescribed a short-acting sleeping medication.

Because of her anxiety issues she was referred to the Cardiology Department, but her ECG and all other investigations proved normal. There was no evidence of caffeine abuse, nor of other drug or alcohol misuse, and no significant problems in terms of her family or social situation. She had been occasionally threatened (thus her emigration) in her old country, but had never suffered any physical abuse.

In the clinic she was smartly groomed, but tended to pick at her fingers nervously. She cried when giving some of her history, and described her mood as worried, depressed and at times hard to describe. She expressed her worries about a possible heart condition, and asked for more help with her regular headaches. She was particularly concerned about having some possible, serious, underlying illness that had been missed, but denied any abnormal experiences, for example panic attacks or memory loss, and showed limited insight into what might be the matter with her.

COMMENTS

None of her investigations had shown any abnormality, including thyroid function tests and various scans. She was considered to have a generalized anxiety disorder, with a mild secondary agoraphobia because of her limited social contacts (she could go out on her own sometimes) and admitted to a dislike of very crowded places. Treatment was centred around an anxiety management approach, using breath control training (she had hyperventilated during the clinic assessment) and detailed advice (pamphlets and tapes) about the nature of her problem (*Box 9.1*). A graded reduction of medication was initiated, aimed at fully discontinuing painkillers, and getting her to take diazepam no more than several times a week. To help with this she was started on an anxiolytic SSRI, and after some 6 months was taking that and only an occasional diazepam (2 mg) several times a week. She continued to use occasional painkillers, but again no more than once or twice a week. She had also been accustomed to drinking 12 or more cups of tea each day, and had managed to reduce this to no more than three or four cups a day.

Although continuing to attend her GP for intermittent minor physical ailments over the next 3 years, her attendance rate reduced by about 70%, and she obtained a part-time job.

9.5 Can obsessive–compulsive disorder (OCD) be distinguished from other neuroses?

Mrs E was a 64-year-old widow, who had become increasingly isolated. Although she maintained contact with her daughter and several other friends, they had found it very difficult to contact her at home, the phone often ringing for 3 or 4 minutes before being answered. She described feeling very depressed and near-suicidal, when consulting her GP, who also noted a dry, red, scaly rash on her hands.

BOX 9.1 Essentials of an anxiety management clinic
1. Being able to assess patients anywhere, e.g. home/day centre/outpatients
2. Good-quality material (tapes, pamphlets, drawings)
3. *Knowing* the physiology and typical symptoms of anxiety states
4. Combining individual and group approaches, on a regular basis
5. Use of relaxation training and/or re-breathing techniques as a first step (like learning to stop when you start skiing)
6. Auditing the results via patient feedback, with recruitment of carers if possible.

On psychiatric assessment she gave a 3-year history of increasing fears about dirt and germs. This had led her to start washing her hands more frequently, after any possible encounter with dirt. This fear of contamination grew to include touching a door handle, a telephone, anything on the floor, and of course anything outside. All shopping expeditions would be followed by a 35-minute ritual of washing her hands, up to the elbows and back like a surgeon, at least three times, in a formal pattern that had to be started again if any mistake was made in the sequence. She was spending up to £40 a week on cleaning products, and often staying up at night hoovering and washing.

Alongside these features she described difficulty sleeping, with early-morning waking and feeling tired in the morning. She worried that she was letting people down, felt tired and anxious during the day, and had lost about half a stone in weight. On examination she came across as a friendly but troubled soul, with clear scarring on her hands as well as markedly dry skin, and she described an intense fear that she was dirty all the time, could smell the dirt, and that unless she carried out her washing rituals these fears would continue to haunt her. Asked to wipe her fingers on the carpet she was completely unable to do so, despite a friendly demonstration by the assessing doctor.

COMMENTS

In view of her depressive and obsessional symptoms she was started on clomipramine, which she tolerated quite well. She was also referred to a clinical psychologist for a behavioural approach, based on encouraging her to touch possibly 'dirty' objects and then helping her to refrain from washing rituals. However, after two home sessions she began to become much more cheerful, and within 3 months of starting medication had ceased her excessive buying of cleansing products. She began answering the phone directly (instead of waiting for it to ring so many times), cut down her hand washing to no more than half a dozen times (single times) a day, and had even decided, eventually, to buy a dog. Over 5 years she has remained entirely stable, in terms of mood and obsessions, on clomipramine 50 mg a day, and has required no additional behaviour therapy input.

9.6 What is a typical case of simple phobia?

Ms F, aged 26, was herself a nurse, and admitted to minor obsessional and anxiety traits. Thus, she would regularly check the oven and electric switches before going to bed, sometimes twice, and was at times a little slow at carrying out her duties because of her concern for things being 'right'. She also found it hard to travel, because as a child she had suffered from travel sickness, and had a distinct fear of being sick.

Offered the chance to go on a sailing trip with her boyfriend, she became very frightened that she would be seasick, but nevertheless wanted to go. Although aware of behaviour therapy approaches, she was a little sceptical, and bet a nurse therapist friend that she could not be helped.

Her friend accepted the challenge, and the two of them went out one evening with three other colleagues for a Chinese meal. They then went to an agreed (and unused) bathroom area in the hospital, and swallowed ipecacuanha. All five vomited over the next 2 hours, in various 'colourful' ways, helped by them all being mildly drunk. Although initially panicky, Ms F was persuaded to stay with the group, noticed her palpitations and anxiety gradually recede, and even found herself laughing at her previous fears.

She went on the boat trip, was only seasick once, but did not end up marrying the boyfriend. Nevertheless she had overcome her generalized fear of travel (secondary to her phobia of vomiting) and has not required any further treatment.

9.7   A typical case of social phobia, or just common shyness?

Mr J was a 55-year-old stores clerk who had taken early retirement on medical grounds. Because of constant anxiety symptoms, he consulted his GP and was prescribed diazepam, which he found made him simply feel rather strange, with little relief of his symptoms.

A fuller history showed that he had been a somewhat solitary individual for much of his life. He had lived with his mother and then alone after her death (some 10 years earlier) and had found it very difficult (in particular) to talk to women, even though he was heterosexual. He was readily tongue-tied, finding he did not know what to say, and found it increasingly hard even to eat in public places. He had tried to join some evening classes, but had found it almost impossible to ask questions or give any kind of presentations, despite there only being half a dozen other members. He was a non-drinker and non-smoker, and since his retirement was spending both his days and evenings alone.

On assessment, he presented a small book outlining his life story, describing himself as a 'social wimp', and listing his various fears. His hopes from treatment included being able to get a girlfriend, being able to feel calmer, and being able to do more. Apart from typical minor panic episodes (e.g. dry mouth, occasional palpitations, sweats) in specific situations, for example meeting a stranger, or having to talk to even two or three people together, there were no other symptoms, although he admitted at times to occasional suicidal ideas.

COMMENTS

Since he had used the term 'depressed', this was acknowledged to him as a form of that condition, and he was treated with an anxiolytic SSRI. He was also referred to the day hospital for a programme of assertiveness training, anxiety management and attendance at open-ended and semi-informal group work. Further social interventions followed on the marked reduction in his social phobic symptoms that occurred over the next 3 months. Thus he served as a volunteer in a shop, went on a computer course at the nearby university, and developed several new friendships.

Follow-up over 5 years on a 6-monthly basis (he described seeing his consultant regularly as a kind of 'insurance') showed good stability of living, no anxiety symptoms, and a wry humour about his past and present situation. He helped write a small pamphlet about panic and anxiety symptoms, from the 'user' point of view, but still does not have a girlfriend.

The Hospital Anxiety and Depression Scale

Doctors are aware that emotions play an important part in most illnesses. If your doctor knows about these feelings, he/she will be able to help you more. This questionnaire is designed to help your doctor to know how you feel. Read each item and circle the score beside the reply which comes closest to how you have been feeling in the past week. Don't take too long over your replies; your immediate reaction to each item will probably be more accurate than a long thought out response.

Circle one score per item

D / A

I feel tense or 'wound up':
3 Most of the time
2 A lot of the time
1 From time to time, occasionally
0 Not at all

I still enjoy the things I used to enjoy:
0 Definitely as much
1 Not quite so much
2 Only a little
3 Hardly at all

I get a sort of frightened feeling as if something awful is about to happen:
3 Very definitely and quite badly
2 Not quite so much now
1 Definitely not so much now
0 Not at all

I can laugh and see the funny side of things:
0 As much as I always could
1 Not quite so much now
2 Definitely not so much now
3 Not at all

Worrying thoughts go through my mind:
3 A great deal of the time
2 A lot of the time
1 From time to time but not too often
0 Only occasionally

I feel cheerful:
3 Not at all
2 Not often
1 Sometimes
0 Most of the time

I can sit at ease and feel relaxed:
0 Definitely
1 Usually
2 Not often
3 Not at all

D / A

I feel as if I am slowed down:
3 Nearly all the time
2 Very often
1 Sometimes
0 Not at all

I get a sort of frightened feeling like 'butterflies' in the stomach:
0 Not at all
1 Occasionally
2 Quite often
3 Very often

I have lost interest in my appearance:
3 Definitely
2 I don't take so much care as I should
1 I may not take quite as much care
0 I take just as much care as ever

I feel restless as if I have to be on the move:
3 Very much indeed
2 Quite a lot
1 Not very much
0 Not at all

I look forward with enjoyment to things:
0 As much as I ever did
1 Rather less than I used to
2 Definitely less than I used to
3 Hardly at all

I get sudden feelings of panic:
3 Very often indeed
2 Quite often
1 Not very often
0 Not at all

I can enjoy a good book or radio or TV programme:
0 Often
1 Sometimes
2 Not often
3 Very seldom

Now check to be sure you have answered all the questions

Total score and grading

Total score: Anxiety ———— Depression ————
Grading: 0–7 Non case   8–10 Borderline case   11+ Case

▲

Fig. A1.1 Hospital Anxiety and Depression Scale (HADS), which is completed by the patient. The scoring system has been added to the questionnaire. (From Zigmond & Snaith 1983, with permission)

Revised impact of event scale

On _____ you experienced _____
     (date)   (life event)

Below is a list of comments made by people after stressful life events.
Please check each item, indicating how frequently these comments
were true for you *DURING THE PAST SEVEN DAYS.*
If they did not occur during that time, please mark the 'Not at all' column.

		FREQUENCY		
	Not at all	Rarely	Sometimes	Often
1. I thought about it when I didn't mean to.	☐	☐	☐	☐
2. I avoided letting myself get upset when I thought about it or was reminded of it.	☐	☐	☐	☐
3. I tried to remove it from memory.	☐	☐	☐	☐
4. I had trouble falling asleep or staying asleep, because of pictures or thoughts about it that came into my mind.	☐	☐	☐	☐
5. I had waves of strong feelings about it.	☐	☐	☐	☐
6. I had dreams about it.	☐	☐	☐	☐
7. I stayed away from reminders of it.	☐	☐	☐	☐
8. I felt as if it hadn't happened or wasn't real.	☐	☐	☐	☐
9. I tried not to talk about it.	☐	☐	☐	☐
10. Pictures of it popped into my mind.	☐	☐	☐	☐
11. Other things kept making me think about it.	☐	☐	☐	☐
12. I was aware that I still had a lot of feelings about it, but I didn't deal with them.	☐	☐	☐	☐
13. I tried not to think about it.	☐	☐	☐	☐
14. Any reminder brought back feelings about it.	☐	☐	☐	☐
15. My feelings about it were kind of numb.	☐	☐	☐	☐

Intrusion subset = 1, 4, 5, 6, 10, 11, 14; avoidance subset = 2, 3, 7, 8, 9, 12, 13, 15

▲

Fig. A1.2 Revised Impact of Event Scale. (From Horowitz et al 1979, with permission)

APPENDIX 2
Useful websites and addresses

FURTHER INFORMATION

Association for Advancement of Behavior Therapy (AABT)

The AABT is a professional, interdisciplinary organization which is concerned with the application of behavioural and cognitive sciences to understanding human behaviour, and developing and promoting empirically supported interventions. It is based in New York, USA.

Website: http://www.aabt.org

BMJ articles

This site provides a collection of recent *BMJ* articles on anxiety disorders, including OCD and PTSD.

Website: http://bmj.com/cgi/collection/anxiety

Centre for Evidence Based Mental Health

Evidence-based mental health site of the Department of Psychiatry of the University of Oxford.

Website: http://www.cebmh.com/

dotCOMSENSE

The American Psychological Association (APA) website. It gives information on how to protect privacy online and assess mental health information on the Internet.

Website: http://www.dotcomsense.com/index.html

Emory Clinical Trials

Website for the mood and anxiety disorders clinical trials at Emory University in Atlanta, Georgia, USA. It offers listings of current research trials for panic disorder, social phobia, OCD, generalized anxiety disorder, and PTSD.

Website: http://www.emoryclinicaltrials.com

Internet Mental Health

A Canadian site for anyone who has an interest in mental health. It provides information on diagnosis, description (European, US), treatment and recent research findings, along with a magazine and links to external sources of information.

Website: http://www.mentalhealth.com/

National Institute of Mental Health (NIMH)
NIMH is based in Bethesda, Maryland, USA. The site offers research reports and up-to-date information on anxiety, panic and related disorders, and their treatment for both practitioners and patients.
Website: http://www.nimh.nih.gov/

National Service Framework for mental health
Website: http://www.doh.gov.uk/nsf/mentalhealth.htm

Primary care Mental Health Education (PriMHE)
A non-profit making organization which aims to help primary health care professionals deliver the best standards of mental health care in various ways, including educational and training initiatives, fostering and sharing of best practice, encouraging research and development, and establishing collaborative and supportive partnerships with all concerned organisations.
Website: http://www.primhe.org/

PsychNet-UK
PsychNet-UK is an independent psychology and mental health information site, run for the benefit of mental health professionals or those interested in mental health practices. It provides disorder information sheets and information on DSM-IV criteria.
Website: http://www.psychnet-uk.com/dsm_iv/dsm_iv_index.htm

Royal College of Psychiatrists
The RCP website provides information on anxiety disorders, including online leaflets and factsheets and information about sources of further help (some of which are included in this list).
Royal College of Psychiatrists
National Headquarters
17 Belgrave Square
London SW1X 8PG
Tel: 020 7235 2351
Fax: 020 7245 1231
Email: rcpsych@rcpsych.ac.uk
Website: http://www.rcpsych.ac.uk/info/index.htm

Social Anxiety Disorder Australia
Providing information, education and support to consumers, carers, health practitioners and the wider community on all aspects of Social Anxiety Disorder.
Website: http://www.socialanxiety.com.au/

WHO Guide to Mental Health in Primary Care

This guide, which was developed by the WHO Collaborating Centre for Research and Training for Mental Health, Institute of Psychiatry, Kings College, London, is designed to help primary care clinicians help people with mental ill health. A brief summary of diagnosis and management is given for each condition and the management summaries include information for the patient, advice and support, descriptions of treatment methods and indications for specialist referrals. They are supported by a linked set of resources: a mental disorder assessment guide; interactive summary cards; and patient information and self-help leaflets.

Website: http://cebmh.warne.ox.ac.uk/cebmh/whoguidemhpcuk/

PATIENT INFORMATION AND SUPPORT

Anxieties.COM

Anxieties.COM is a self-help source for people with anxiety, panic attacks, OCD, fear of flying, and other phobias. It includes medication issues and offers books and tapes for sale. The site is by psychologist/psychiatrist R. Reid Wilson, PhD, and is based in Chapel Hill, North Carolina, USA.

Website: http://www.anxieties.com

Anxiety Care

Anxiety Care is a charity based in East London that specializes in helping people to recover from anxiety disorder through personal recovery programmes based on self-help and supported by skilled volunteers.

Anxiety Care
Cardinal Heenan Centre
326 High Road
Ilford
Essex IG1 1QP
Tel: (020) 8262 8891/2
Helpline: (020) 8478 3400
Email: anxietycare@aol.com
Website: http://www.anxietycare.org.uk/

Anxiety Network International

The Anxiety Network, which is based in Phoenix, Arizona, USA, provides information on social anxiety disorder (social phobia), panic, and generalized anxiety disorder. The site, by Thomas A. Richards, PhD, includes a social anxiety mailing list, chat room, bookstore, question and answer pages, and related links.

Website: http://www.anxietynetwork.com/

Anxiety Panic Hub

This is an Australian site offering information on anxiety disorders, including frequently asked questions, and both online and one-to-one telephone support for those affected.

Panic & Anxiety Hub
PO Box 516
Goolwa
South Australia 5214
Tel/fax: 0 8 8555 5012 (Australian residents); 61 8 8555 5012 (International)
Email: hub@panicattacks.com.au
Website: http://www.panicattacks.com.au/

Anxiety/Panic Attack Resource Site

This American site offers help to those who suffer from anxiety/panic attacks, by providing support and information on medications, treatments and symptoms.

Website: http://anxietypanic.com

Connects

Connects is a free, linking website for mental health in general. It contains information about organizations, websites, events, and news items concerned with mental health or learning disabilities.

Website: http://www.connects.org.uk

Facts For Health

Facts for Health is a comprehensive resource to help identify, understand and treat a number of important medical conditions; including aspects of social anxiety and PTSD. It was created by Drs Greist, Jefferson and Katzelnick of the Madison Institute of Medicine, Madison, Wisconsin, USA.

Website: http://factsforhealth.org

First Steps to Freedom

First Steps to Freedom is a UK charity which aims to provide practical help for people who suffer from phobias, OCD, general anxiety, panic attacks, anorexia and bulimia and those who wish to come off tranquillizers, together with help for their carers. It offers practical advice, a telephone helpline, telephone self-help groups and one-to-one counselling, leaflets, self-help booklets, videotapes and audiotapes.

Helpline: +44 (0)1926 851608
Website: http://www.first-steps.org/

Freedom From Fear (FFF)

FFF is an American mental health advocacy association founded in 1984 by Mary Guardino and based on Staten Island, New York. It provides aid and counselling for individuals and their families who suffer from anxiety and depression.

Website: http://www.freedomfromfear.com

Medical Foundation for the Care of Victims of Torture

The Medical Foundation for the Care of Victims of Torture is a UK charity that provides survivors of torture with medical treatment, practical assistance and psychotherapeutic support.

Website: http://www.torturecare.org.uk/

Mental Health Foundation

The Mental Health Foundation is a UK charity working in the fields of mental health and learning disabilities. Its publications include newsletters, books/booklets and factsheets on mental health issues.

Mental Health Foundation
UK Office
7th Floor, 83 Victoria Street
London SW1H 0HW
Tel: + 44 (0) 20 7802 0300
Fax: + 44 (0) 20 7802 0301
Email: mhf@mhf.org.uk
Scotland Office
5th Floor, Merchants House
30 George Square
Glasgow G2 1EG
Tel: + 44 (0) 141 572 0125
Fax: + 44 (0) 141 572 0246
Email: scotland@mhf.org.uk
Website: http://www.mentalhealth.org.uk

Mental Help Net

This American 'megasite' is a comprehensive source of online mental health information, news and resources.

Website: http://mentalhelp.net/

Mind

Mind is a mental health charity in England and Wales which works for everyone in emotional distress, campaigning for rights and developing locally based services. Mind's national information line covers all aspects of mental health, including legal matters for service users, carers, family and friends, researchers, students, service providers and the public. Mind publishes a bi-monthly magazine and has a free quarterly newsletter as well as many other publications.

Mind
Granta House
15–19 Broadway
Stratford
London E15 4BQ
Tel: + 44 (0) 20 8519 2122
Mind Information Line: + 44 (0) 20 8522 1728 (Greater London) or + 44 (0) 8457 660 163 (elsewhere) (9.15 a.m. – 4.45 p.m. Mon., Wed. and Thurs.)
Email: contact@mind.org.uk
Website: http://www.mind.org.uk

National Phobics Society

NPS is a national charity for those affected by anxiety disorders; it is run by sufferers and ex-sufferers and supported by a panel of medical advisors. Membership services include an online chat room and bulletin board, a telephone helpline and specialist phone-in sessions, factsheets, information booklets and a quarterly newsletter, and a national network of self-help groups.

National Phobics Society
Zion Community Resource Centre
339 Stretford Road
Hulme
Manchester M15 4ZY
Tel: 0870 7700 456
Fax: 0161 227 9862
Email: natphob.soc@good.co.uk
Website: http://www.phobics-society.org.uk/

No Panic

No Panic is a charity, whose aims are to aid the relief and rehabilitation of people suffering from panic attacks, phobias, OCD and other related anxiety disorders, including tranquillizer withdrawal, and to support them and their families and/or carers. Services offered include a helpline, pop-in centres, telephone recovery groups and one-to-one telephone mentoring, a contact booklet for phone- and pen-friends, leaflets, audio and video cassettes, and a written recovery programme (self-help, based on cognitive and behaviour therapy).

No Panic
93 Brands Farm Way

Telford
Shropshire TF3 2JQ
Tel: + 44 (0) 1952 590005 (office)
Helpline: + 44 (0) 1952 590545 (10 a.m.– 10 p.m. every day)
Freephone: + 44 (0) 800 783 1531 (information line only – answerphone)
Fax: +44 (0) 1952 270962
Email colin.hammond@no-panic.co.uk
Website: http://www.no-panic.co.uk/

Obsessive Action

Obsessive Action is a charity established to help people experiencing OCD and to advance awareness, research, understanding and treatment of the disorder. Members receive regular newsletters and information bulletins and are able to attend conferences and open-days. Factsheets on effective treatments and recommended reading are also available.

Obsessive Action
Aberdeen Centre
22–24 Highbury Grove
London N5 2EA
Tel: + 44 (0) 20 7226 4000 Mon/Wed/Fri (not helpline)
Email: admin@obsessive-action.demon.co.uk
Website: http://www.obsessive-action.demon.co.uk

Obsessive–Compulsive Foundation (OCF)

The OCF is an international non-profit-making organization, based in North Branford, Connecticut, USA. It is composed of people with OCD and related disorders, their families, friends, professionals and other concerned individuals.

Website: http://www.ocfoundation.org

Panic Center

This Canadian site, based in Toronto, Ontario, aims to promote communication between people with panic disorder and health care professionals. It offers an anxiety screening test, an interactive diary, an online CBT programme and a moderated support group.

Website: http://www.paniccenter.net

Panic Disorder Institute (PDI)

The Panic Disorder Institute, director Stuart Shipko, MD, is based in Pasadena, California, USA. The site explores the medicine and psychology of panic disorder, answers frequently asked questions, and hosts a discussion group.

Website: http://www.algy.com/pdi

Pax

Pax offers an information and advisory service for people who suffer from panic attacks, agoraphobia, social and other related phobias, and anxiety problems. Books, cassettes and a bi-monthly newsletter are available. Send a stamped addressed envelope for a free information pack.

Pax
4 Manorbrook
Blackheath
London SE3 9AW
Tel: + 44 (0) 20 8318 5026
Website: http://www.panicattacks.co.uk

Phobic Action

Phobic Action offers practical self-help to people affected by anxiety, and their carers.

Phobic Action
Claybury Grounds
Manor Road
Woodford Green
Essex IG8 8PR
Tel: + 44 (0) 20 8559 2551 (office)
Helpline: + 44 (0) 20 8559 2459

Samaritans

The Samaritans offer a confidential 24-hour helpline for anyone in the UK experiencing emotional distress. Details of local branches can be found in a local telephone directory.

The Samaritans
10 The Grove
Slough
Berks SL1 1QP
National helpline: + 44 (0) 345 909090
Website: http://www.samaritans.org.uk

SANE

SANE is a campaigning mental health charity. Its helpline, SANELINE, gives information and support to anyone coping with mental illness.

SANE
2nd Floor, Worthington House
199–205 Old Marylebone Road
London W1 5QP
Tel: + 44 (0) 20 7375 1002 (office)
SANELINE: + 44 (0) 845 767 8000 (open from 12 noon until 2 a.m. every

day of the year)
Website: http://www.sane.org.uk

SA-UK

SA-UK is a site for people with social anxiety, run by people with social anxiety. It provides information on SA and external links to other sources of information and support, including a list of local self-help groups. It also aims to promote meetings and events, and to raise the profile of social anxiety.

SA-UK
PO Box 5283
Burton-On-Trent
Staffs DE15 0ZD
Website: http://www.social-anxiety.org.uk/

Scottish Association for Mental Health

The Scottish Association for Mental Health provides an information service and leaflets on general mental health issues.

Scottish Association for Mental Health
Cumbrae House
15 Carlton Court
Glasgow G5 9JP
Tel: +44 (0) 141 568 7000
Email: enquire@samh.org.uk
Website: http://www.samh.org.uk

Stress Management Training Institute

The SMTI offers a wide range of materials and training courses to help reduce stress.

SMTI
'Foxhills'
30 Victoria Avenue
Shanklin
Isle of Wight PO37 6LS
Tel: 01983 868 166

Stress Watch Scotland

Stress Watch Scotland is a voluntary organization which supports people suffering from stress, anxiety, phobias, panic attacks and OCD. In addition to providing a telephone helpline and recovery group, it gives guidance in setting up self-help groups in Scotland.

Stress Watch Scotland
The Barn
42 Barnwell Road

Kilmarnock KA1 4JF
Tel: + 44 (0) 1563 574144
Website: http://web.ukonline.co.uk/members/stresswatch.scotland/

Thanet Phobic Group
The Thanet Phobic Group helps with the rehabilitation of stressed and phobic people by giving moral support.

Thanet Phobic Group
47 Orchard Rd
Westbrook
Margate
Kent CT9 5JS
Tel: 01843 833 720

the Anxiety Panic internet resource (tAPir) (USA)
tAPir is an American self-help site run by volunteers, with an emphasis on information and support for people with anxiety disorders. It answers frequently asked questions on anxiety and panic, and provides a bulletin board and updated headlines.

Website: http://www104.pair.com/algy/anxiety/anxiety.html

Triumph Over Phobia (TOP UK)
TOP UK runs a national network of 16 structured self-help groups, run by trained lay volunteers, for sufferers of phobias or OCD. Information on local groups can be obtained by sending a stamped addressed envelope to head office.

Triumph Over Phobia (TOP UK)
PO Box 1831
Bath BA1 3XY
Tel: + 44 (0) 1225 330353 (admin. line)
Email: triumphoverphobia@compuserve.com
Website: http://www.triumphoverphobia.com

REFERENCES

Chapter 1

Beers M H, Berkow R (eds) 1999 The Merck manual of diagnosis and therapy, 17th edn. Merck, Whitehouse Station NJ

Ferriman A 2001 Levels of neurosis remained static in the 1990s. British Medical Journal 323: 130

Hale, A 1998 Anxiety. In: Davies T, Craig T (eds) ABC of mental health. BMJ Books, London, Ch 6, pp 19–22

World Health Organization 1992 ICD-10 Classification of mental and behavioural disorders. WHO, Geneva

Yerkes R M, Dodson J D 1908 The relation of strength of stimulus to rapidity of habit formation. Journal of Comparative Neurology and Psychology 18:459–482

Yonkers K 1994 Panic disorder in women. Journal of Women's Health 3(6):481–486

Chapter 2

Puri B, Laking P, Treasaden I 1996 Textbook of psychiatry. Churchill Livingstone, London

Chapter 3

Mayon R, Farmer A 2002 ABC of psychological medicine: functional somatic symptoms and syndromes. British Medical Journal 325:265

Chapter 7

Gill D, Bass C 1997 Somatoform and dissociative disorders: assessment and treatment. Advances in Psychiatric Treatment 3:9–16

Mayou R, Farmer A 2002 ABC of psychological medicine: functional somatic symptoms and syndromes. British Medical Journal 325:265–268

Chapter 8

Roy-Byrne P, Katon W, Cowley D et al (2001) A randomized effectiveness trial of collaborative care for patients with panic disorder in primary care. Archives of General Psychiatry 58:869–876

Tyrer P 2001 The case for cothymia: mixed anxiety and depression as a single diagnosis. British Journal of Psychiatry 179:191–193

Appendix 1

Horowitz M, Wilner N, Alvarez W 1979 Impact of Event Scale: a measure of subjective stress. Psychosomatic Medicine 41(3):209–218

Zigmond A S, Snaith R P 1983 The hospital anxiety and depression scale. Acta Psychiatrica Scandinavica 67:361–370

Glossary

Goldberg D, Huxley P 1980 Mental illness in the community, the pathway to psychiatric care. Tavistock Publications, London

FURTHER READING

GENERAL TEXTS

Useful descriptions of the anxiety disorders and their management can be found in standard textbooks. Two of the most readable are:

Gelder M, Mayou R, Geddes J 1998 Psychiatry – an Oxford core text, 2nd edn. Oxford, University Press, Oxford

Puri B, Laking P, Treasaden I 2002 Textbook of psychiatry, 2nd edn. Churchill Livingstone, Edinburgh

A more academic text summarizing modern research is:

Stein G, Wilkinson G (eds) 1998 Seminars in general adult psychiatry. Royal College of Psychiatrists/Gaskell Publications, London, vol 1

For treatments overall the most comprehensive resource is:

Andrews C, Jenkins R (eds) 1999 The management of mental disorders, UK edn. WHO Collaborating Centre for Mental Health and Substance Abuse, Sydney

For evidence-based treatments, there is now a specific publication called *Evidence-based Mental Health*. It is published quarterly by the BMJ Publishing Group, and is available online at: http://www.ebmentalhealth. com

It essentially selects and abstracts journal articles, generally down to one page of text, with a commentary that is also succinct and backed up by references. There are usually a number of abstracts around depression/anxiety/panic and their understanding and treatment.

SPECIALIST TEXTS

The following are recommended for those wishing to read further:

Nutt, D, Ballenger J, Lépine J-P (eds) 1999 Panic disorder: clinical diagnosis, management and mechanisms. Martin Dunitz, London

Snaith P 1981 Clinical neurosis. Oxford University Press, Oxford

SPECIFIC ISSUES WITHIN THE OVERALL CONTEXT OF ANXIETY DISORDERS

Books

Davies T, Craig T (eds) 1998 ABC of mental health. BMJ Books, London

See especially:

Ch. 6: Anxiety (Hale A), pp 19–22

Ch. 9: Disorders of personality (Marlowe M, Sugarman P), pp 31–34
Ch. 19: Psychological treatments (Richardson P), pp 72–74

Mayou R, Sharpe M, Carson A (eds) 2002 ABC of psychological medicine, BMJ Books, London

This is an excellent collection of articles on the recognition and management of psychosomatic disorders such as irritable bowel syndrome, fibromyalgia and chronic pain states.

Articles

Alcohol

UK Alcohol Forum 2001 Guidelines for the management of alcohol problems in primary care and general psychiatry, 2nd edn. Tangent Medical Education, London. Online. Available: http://www.ukalcoholforum.org

Anxiety control

Snaith P 1994 Anxiety control training. Advances in Psychiatric Treatment 1:57–61

Assessment

Sundin E, Horowitz M 2002 Impact of Event Scale: psychometric properties. British Journal of Psychiatry 180:205–209

Cognitive behavioural therapy

Williams C, Garland A 2002 A cognitive-behavioural therapy assessment model for use in everyday clinical practice. Advances in Psychiatric Treatment 8:172–179

Diagnosis

Tyrer P 2001 The case for cothymia: mixed anxiety and depression as a single diagnosis. British Journal of Psychiatry 179:191–193

General management

Lader M, Beaumont G, Bond A et al (1992) Guidelines for the management of patients with generalised anxiety. Psychiatric Bulletin 16:560–565

Problem solving in general practice

Catalan J, Gath D, Anastasiades P et al (1991) Evaluation of a brief psychological treatment for emotional disorders in primary care. Psychological Medicine 21:1013–1018

Somatization

Gill D, Bass C 1997 Somatoform and dissociative disorders: assessment and treatment. Advances in Psychiatric Treatment 3:9–16
Salmon P, Peters S, Stanley I 1999 Patients' perceptions of medical explanations for somatisation disorders: quantitative analysis. British Medical Journal 318:372–376

Treatments

Gale C, Oakley-Browne M 2000 Anxiety disorder – extracts from 'clinical evidence'. British Medical Journal 321:1204–1207

Lingford-Hughes A, Potokan J, Nutt D 2002 Treating anxiety complicated by substance misuse. Advances in Psychiatric Treatment 8:107–116

Marks I 2002 The maturing of therapy. Some brief psychotherapies help anxiety/depressive disorder but mechanisms of action are unclear. British Journal of Psychiatry 180:200–204

Nutt D, Bell C 1997 Practical pharmacotherapy for anxiety. Advances in Psychiatric Treatment 3:79–85

Scott A, Davidson A, Palmer K 2001 Antidepressant drugs in the treatment of anxiety disorders. Advances in Psychiatric Treatment 7:275–282

SELF-HELP RESOURCES

Books

Breton S 1996 Don't panic: a guide to overcoming panic attacks. Century Vermilion, London

Kennerley H 1997 Overcoming anxiety. Robinson, London

Marks I 1995 Living with fear. McGraw Hill, New York

Mind 2000 How to cope with panic attacks. Mind, London

Mind 2000 How to cope with sleep problems. Mind, London

Mind 2001 How to stop worrying. Mind, London

Priest R 1996 Anxiety and depression. Century Vermilion, London

Rachman S, de Silva P 1996 Panic disorders – the facts. Oxford University Press, Oxford

Silove D, Manicavasagar V 1997 Overcoming panic. Robinson, London

Weekes C 1995 Peace from nervous suffering. Thorsons, London

Weekes C 1995 Self-help for your nerves. Thorsons, London

Tapes

Control your tension. Lifeskills, Bowman House, 6 Billetfield, Taunton, Somerset TA1 3NN

The Mitchell method of relaxation. Laura Mitchell, 8 Gainsborough Gardens, London NW3 1BJ

GLOSSARY

Affect – A patient's mood or emotional state, as it comes across to the outside observer. Thus the term 'mood' describes subjective experience ('my feelings are…'), whereas the objective description ('affect') can be considered as how it 'affects' other people.

Agoraphobia – An intense fear of crowded places, literally the 'marketplace' (*agora* = Greek for the market), usually caused by panic attacks and leading to avoidance. It is not a fear of 'open' spaces.

Anxiolytic – A drug, prescribed or recreational, or other form of treatment, that relieves anxiety symptoms.

BAI – Beck Anxiety Inventory, a standard checklist using self-report to measure a person's anxiety level.

CBT – Cognitive behavioural therapy, a time-limited, structured psychological intervention, based on assessing and restructuring cognitions (the way one thinks) as well as behaviour.

Conversion – A process whereby psychological anxiety is unconsciously 'converted' into a physical symptom or sign (e.g. loss of speech, loss of feeling in a limb). It is a theoretical description, awaiting a physiological explanation.

Delusion – An abnormal belief, usually false and often bizarre, that dominates one's mind, is not susceptible to reasoned argument, and does not fit with a patient's social or cultural background.

Delusional mood – A state of perplexed anxiety, lasting for days or weeks, that often precedes the brainwave-like impact of a full delusion. It is a differential diagnosis for anxiety states, and characteristic of schizophrenic illnesses.

Depersonalization – A common, but difficult to describe, state of feeling unreal and/or not in touch with the world around one. Typical in panic or anxiety states, it is described as like a veil between the patient and the world, or as if one is in a dream or changed in some way.

Dissociation – This describes the notion of a disconnection between the various aspects of one's psychological make-up. Patients forget who they are (dissociative amnesia), they seem to be in a stupor, or (rarely) develop another personality.

Dyskinesia – A general term to describe movement disorder, of whatever cause, including tics, tremors, and various repetitive limb or body movements.

Dysthymia – The opposite of euthymia, that is a chronic state of mild depression, of a fluctuating nature, that usually does not progress to a full-blown depressive illness, although may do so in older people.

GABA – Gamma-aminobutyric acid, one of the most important inhibitory (i.e. damping-down) transmitters in the central nervous system. The mildest reduction in GABA-ergic activity leads to anxiety, restlessness and arousal; thus the effectiveness of benzodiazepines (which stimulate GABA) in reducing anxiety.

GAD – Generalized anxiety disorder, the *ICD-10* term for what was 'anxiety neurosis'. It is characterized by persisting anxiety, over weeks/months, that includes apprehension, motor tension and autonomic overactivity (e.g. sweating, dry mouth).

GH – Growth hormone, one of the pituitary hormones regulating growth, levels of which are often used in biological research into depression and anxiety.

GHQ – General Health Questionnaire, a widely used symptom checklist, developed in the 1970s, to detect psychiatric illnesses in general practice populations. It was the basis of *Mental Illness in the Community, the Pathway to Psychiatric Care*, by Goldberg & Huxley (1980), one of the most influential publications in the development of psychiatric care.

HADS – Hospital Anxiety and Depression Scale (see Appendix 1) enabling patients to self-rate in terms of symptoms, and thus a useful diagnostic and treatment tool.

Hallucination – A perception in the absence of a stimulus, in any of the five sensory modalities (taste, touch, smell, sight, hearing) and occurring in clear consciousness. A true hallucination should seem absolutely real to the patient (i.e. hearing voices) and should not be muddled with misinterpretations or illusions, where something really is heard, seen or felt, but whose nature is misjudged (e.g. a shadow in a curtain is mistaken as a face).

MAOI – Monoamine oxidase inhibitor, a group of drugs with antidepressant and anxiety-relieving properties, that work by blocking the enzyme that breaks down certain neurochemicals, e.g. noradrenaline. Their use is limited by dietary requirements and a number of drug interactions.

MMSE – Mini-mental State Examination, a standardized 30-point questionnaire, designed to assess the degree of cognitive impairment. Scoring fewer than 27 (out of 30) generally indicates a degree of brain damage and/or dementia.

OCD – Obsessive–compulsive disorder, a neurosis characterized by persisting obsessions – thoughts that come unbidden into one's mind, that one knows to be probably untrue or unimportant, but which one cannot put out of one's mind. To relieve anxiety, patients resort to compulsive rituals (e.g. hand washing), leading to considerable problems in social function.

Pseudo-hallucination – A term describing an apparent hallucination (see above), for example hearing voices, into which the patient has insight. Thus, the voice is known not to be real, comes from inside one's head, and can be eliminated by effort or distraction.

PTSD – Post-traumatic stress disorder, a condition brought on after a major, usually life-threatening trauma, and characterized by enhanced anxiety, emotional withdrawal, and intrusive thoughts and nightmares (including 'flashbacks') of the accident.

SADS – Seasonal affective disorder syndrome, a type of depression associated with reduced daylight in winter months. More prevalent in northern latitudes, its status is uncertain but individual responses to light therapy can be significant.

Somatization – The tendency to experience physical distress and symptoms that have no organic or pathological basis. The formal category of 'somatization disorder' requires at least 2 years of multiple symptoms, refusal to accept reassurance, and a degree of impaired social functioning.

Somatoform disorder – This term embraces the group of conditions (including 'somatization') that lead patients to repeatedly present with physical symptoms. Patients demand repeated investigations, reject psychological interventions, and are a considerable burden on health services. Pain states, degrees of depression and anxiety, hypochondriasis, and chronic bowel/cardiac/locomotor problems are the typical presentations.

SSRI –Specific serotonin reuptake inhibitor, a relatively new group of antidepressant medications that affect levels of serotonin (also known as 5-HT – 5-hydroxytriptamine) in the brain. Apart from nausea, side-effects are usually much less distressing than those of tricyclic antidepressants. They also have a role in anxiety and obsessional disorders.

State anxiety – This defines the kind of anxiety that comes on at a particular time, for a particular reason, and then resolves. It is a typical response, for example, to a job interview or public performance, such as giving a speech.

TATT – A non-official, but understandable medical shorthand for 'tired all the time'. It has no diagnostic significance, but is the typical presentation of many patients with anxiety and depressive disorders.

Trait anxiety – This characterizes the anxiety-prone personality, with a life-long tendency to be anxious, whatever the surrounding situation. Terms like 'a born worrier', or 'suffering from nerves' often reflect this condition.

Transference – A term derived from Freudian psychoanalytic theory, to describe the way patients often treat a therapist (whether psychotherapist, psychologist or doctor) as they would a parent or sibling. Recognizing this process can be helpful in understanding the basis to their problems.

Tricyclics – A general term to describe a group of antidepressants that have a three-ring structure, such as amitriptyline and imipramine, and have been available for over 40 years now. They are effective antidepressants, and can also be used to treat anxiety and panic states, limitations being their side-effect profile, particularly in older patients.

Trismus – A term describing the tendency to clench one's jaw and/or grind one's teeth, particularly at night when one is asleep. It may present with jaw or teeth problems, or even headaches, and is a not uncommon symptom of anxiety states.

LIST OF PATIENT QUESTIONS

INDEX